YOURSELF

FIT

SIMPLE STEPS TO
A HEALTHIER YOU

Christina Macdonald

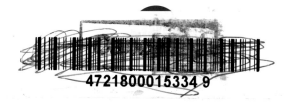

RUN YOURSELF FIT

Vie Books is an imprint of Summersdale Publishers Ltd

Summersdale Publishers Ltd
46 West Street
Chichester
West Sussex
PO19 1RP
UK

www.summersdale.com

Printed and bound in the Czech Republic

ISBN: 978-1-84953-799-5

Substantial discounts on bulk quantities of Summersdale books are available to corporations, professional associations and other organisations. For details contact Nicky Douglas by telephone: +44 (0) 1243 756902, fax: +44 (0) 1243 786300 or email: nicky@summersdale.com.

*For Cheryl Mayhew, who knew I could do it,
and Eddie Macdonald, who made sure I did*

CONTENTS

ACKNOWLEDGEMENTS

Alzheimer's Society; Asthma UK; Blood Pressure UK; British Heart Foundation; Cancer Research UK; Lifetime Training; Mind; National Osteoporosis Society; Tim Allardyce, physiotherapist; Mark Buckingham, physiotherapist; Tim Elsey, assistant manager, Runners Need; Gert van der Walt, chiropractor.

Extended thanks:
Nick Anderson, running coach at www.runningwithus.com; Christine Bailey, nutritionist; Sarah Ellis, nutritional therapist; Mark Hatfield, personal trainer; Stuart Mailer, physiotherapist; Jonathan Quint, EMEA marketing manager, Saucony.

So unless you looked like an athlete training for a serious sporting event, you might have felt a tad uneasy while pounding the streets. Fortunately, things have now changed for the better. Nowadays, people of all shapes and sizes choose to run. The increase in mass-participation events has led to a huge surge in its popularity in the past ten years, with many people keen to raise money for charity or wanting to set an achievable fitness goal.

As an exercise choice, running is cheap compared with other sports and fitness regimes (you need only minimal kit), as well as being convenient and adaptable. You can do it anywhere in the world; there's no need to pay for a gym membership; you can run when it suits you, making it easy to fit into a busy routine; you can vary your route or stay indoors and run on a treadmill; or, you can make it a social activity, either by joining a local running group or by getting involved in fun runs.

It's also an activity that requires minimal coordination – you don't need to learn fancy choreography – as all you need to do is put one foot in front of the other.

So it's no surprise that running is now considered a natural exercise choice for the masses. Not only that, but the health benefits are significant, and when you read about them (see chapter 1), you'll want to make running a regular part of your life.

As a new runner, this book will give you all the information and advice you need to start running and improve. From choosing the right kit to building stamina gradually and getting prepared for your first race, *Run Yourself Fit* has everything you need to take those first steps, building up confidence and fitness at your own pace.

So if you want to improve your health, slim your waistline and boost your self-esteem, you've picked the right exercise to achieve all of those things and so much more.

Christina Macdonald
September 2015

" I love the feeling of freedom when I run. The freedom for my mind to think and for my body to move. "

NELL McANDREW, BUSY MUM, MARATHON RUNNER

Chapter 1

HEALTH AND LONGEVITY

Hands up who wants to be slimmer, fitter, feel more confident, have a healthier heart, enjoy a better quality of life and live longer? Running will help you burn fat, lose weight and maintain a healthy body weight. It's estimated to burn around 10 to 15 calories per minute, depending on your age, weight, average running speed and current fitness levels. So, if combined with a healthy diet, it will help with weight loss and appearance. Many people initially start running to lose weight but, interestingly, the more you run, the less important weight loss becomes and the more you begin to appreciate the wider benefits.

RUN FOR A HEALTHY HEART

Regular running will reduce your risk of heart disease and extend your lifespan. An international study conducted by the American Medical Association showed that running could extend your life by up to three and a half years. Some studies have even shown an increase in life expectancy of up to seven years.

Running will significantly improve your heart health: it provides the ideal workout and is an effective way to strengthen it. When demands are made on muscle fibres, they respond by thickening and strengthening themselves. Over time, this means heart rate can actually reduce as, due to its increased capacity, the heart does not have to work so hard.

Running also helps lower blood pressure, and reduce cholesterol and diabetes risk, all of which are factors for heart disease.

RUN TO LIVE LONGER

Running is beneficial for older people. Professor James Fries of Stanford University in California looked at runners' heart health over an extensive period of 20 years and found that older runners were at less risk of heart disease than their peers.

Being regularly active will help you remain healthy and give you a better quality of life in later years. According to the World Health Organization (WHO), a sedentary lifestyle is one of ten leading causes of death and disability. It is also a primary risk factor for a variety of diseases, such as arthritis, obesity, certain cancers, heart disease and stroke. The WHO lists the benefits of being physically active as follows:

- Reduced risk of premature death
- Reduced risk of coronary heart disease by 40 per cent
- Reduced risk of stroke by 20 to 40 per cent
- Reduced risk of Type 2 diabetes by 30 per cent
- Reduced risk of hip fracture by 40 per cent
- Reduced risk of falling by 10 to 20 per cent
- Reduced risk of breast cancer in women by 30 per cent
- Reduced risk of dementia by around 30 per cent *

WHO statistics provided by Lifetime Training (www.lifetimetraining.co.uk)

* Alzheimer's Society

RUN TO REDUCE BLOOD PRESSURE

Regular running will help reduce your blood pressure and keep it in the healthy range (a healthy reading is around 120/80). According to the charity Blood Pressure UK, around 16 million people in England have high blood pressure – or around 31 per cent of males and 28 per cent of females.

If you have high blood pressure or cardiovascular disease, the British Heart Foundation (www.bhf.org.uk) recommends speaking to your GP before you start running, as well as building up gradually and following your GP's instructions once you have the all clear.

RUN TO REDUCE RISK OF DISEASES

Regular cardiovascular exercise like running can decrease your risk of developing certain cancers. Cancer Research UK says that regular exercise can prevent bowel cancer by increasing the rate at which food moves through our bowels. This reduces the amount of time that the lining of the bowel is in contact with any harmful chemicals, like those released through the consumption of red or processed meats, or alcohol. The end result is that there's less chance of them being able to cause damage that could lead to cancer.

Another way that exercise can prevent cancer is by helping reduce the amount of insulin in our blood. Scientists think that insulin can turn on signals that tell cells to multiply. Cancer starts when cells multiply out of control, so reducing insulin levels could help stop some types of cancer from developing. Cancer Research UK has also stated that there is good evidence that being active can help people during and after cancer treatment. TV talk show host Trisha Goddard is a testament to that. She continued her running while having radiotherapy treatment for breast cancer. She even ran to her radiotherapy sessions. Incidentally, she is now cancer-free.

RUN FOR A HEALTHY MIND

Running is also hugely beneficial for your mental health. According to the mental health charity Mind, regular cardiovascular exercise like running can be more effective at treating mild to moderate depression than taking antidepressants. When you exercise, your anxiety levels will drop and your mood will improve. You may feel a reduction in stress levels and you'll also be able to think more clearly. As you gain confidence through your running, your self-esteem will increase, which can also reduce the likelihood of feeling depressed. Mind has stated that switching from a sedentary lifestyle to doing some cardiovascular exercise at least three times per week can reduce your risk of depression by up to 20 per cent. Outdoor runs can be ideal for lifting mood. 'The colours, sounds and smells of the great outdoors stimulate our senses in a way that the gym or urban environments don't,' says Mind press officer Camilla Swain from the charity Mind. 'This can help relieve stress and clear our heads of day-to-day pressure.'

There's strong evidence to show that regular cardiovascular exercise like running can also help reduce your risk of developing dementia. Dementia, a brain condition that currently affects 850,000 people in the UK, causes memory loss and confusion. The number of sufferers is expected to rise to over one million by 2025. Alzheimer's Society has been looking at several studies on middle-aged people and the effects of physical exercise, like running, on their thinking and memory in later life. Combining the results of 11 studies shows that regular exercise can significantly reduce the risk of developing dementia by about 30 per cent. The risk of Alzheimer's disease (the most common type of dementia) was reduced by 45 per cent. Older people can also benefit from exercise for brain health. In a study of 716 people with an average age of 82 years, people in the bottom ten per cent in terms of the amount of their daily physical activity were more than twice as likely to develop Alzheimer's disease as those in the top ten per cent. In a modest-sized clinical trial, one year of aerobic (cardiovascular) exercise showed a small increase in the size of the hippocampus (the key brain area involved in memory). This was the equivalent to reversing one to two years of age-related shrinkage.

RUN FOR BETTER BONES

The list of benefits continues. According to the National Osteoporosis Society (NOS), running is one form of weight-bearing exercise that can help maintain and improve bone strength. (Weight-bearing exercise means any exercise where you are supporting your own body weight.) The NOS says it's an effective way of loading your bones and strengthening them, therefore reducing the risks of fractures.

RUN FOR BETTER SLEEP

Running can improve sleep quality, and sleep is essential for our bodies to repair themselves. Sleep can also reduce the rate at which our minds age. In a study published by the website *ScienceDaily*, evidence suggests that those who sleep less than 6 to 8 hours per night are subject to accelerated cognitive decline. Other studies indicate that poor sleep may speed up the onset of age-related conditions such as Type 2 diabetes, high blood pressure and memory loss. A study published in the *Journal of Clinical Sleep Medicine* took a small group of sedentary, older adults with insomnia and made them do aerobic exercise, like running, for 16 weeks, three times a week. By the end of the 16-week period, they were getting an extra 45 minutes of sleep per night compared with another group not doing any exercise.

So the evidence is compelling – regular running will extend your life and reduce your risk of disease. With all of these benefits, combined with the fact that it's cheap and convenient, it's definitely worth giving it a try. Approach it with an open mind and a positive attitude and you'll soon feel fitter and healthier. And if you're already running, you've got some great reasons to keep doing it.

AT A GLANCE

- Running can extend your lifespan
- Running can reduce your risk of dementia, osteoporosis, heart disease, stroke and certain cancers, and can improve joint health
- Running can improve your mental well-being by releasing 'feel-good' endorphins
- Running can help you sleep better

" I run for my head. My feet marking time to my favourite music is better than clubbing because you're your own DJ and your shoes are way more comfortable. Plus the runner's high is cheaper than booze! "

TRISHA GODDARD, TV PRESENTER, RECREATIONAL RUNNER

Chapter 2

YOUR QUESTIONS ANSWERED

You know the benefits of running, but you may have heard some negative comments that have left you with a few nagging doubts. You may have listened to people say that it will harm your joints, make your boobs sag, cause nasty chafing or make you wet yourself, none of which will motivate you to get started. So let's tackle some common misconceptions first…

WILL RUNNING AFFECT MY JOINTS?

Running is a high-impact activity. When you run, a force equal to approximately two and a half to three times your bodyweight will go through your knees (the exact amount depends on strength, speed and running technique). Although this sounds like you are subjecting your body to a lot of excess weight and stress, research suggests that some loading of the joints can be good for us.

While you don't have to be thin to run, it also stands to reason that if you're carrying excess weight, the shock forces will be greater, subjecting your body to more stress. But you don't need to be a certain size to run and running is an ideal way to lose weight, making it a good choice for those who are overweight.

'Running can improve our joint and bone health, especially if we manage the volume and frequency of our runs,' says physiotherapist Stuart Mailer. 'When we run there is a high stress and load going through our joints and bone tissue that can improve bone density, helping prevent osteoporosis and osteoarthritis. This is because the bone remodels itself frequently and adapts to the stress it is put through. So running can help our joint health so long as we are sensible with regards to our fitness levels, age, volume and intensity.'

However, not everyone is suited to running long distances, like marathons for example. It appears that we inherit the quality of our cartilage and joint health from our parents. More research is needed on the link between genetics and joint health, but it is currently believed that we produce different amounts of collagen, which is part of the connective tissues (including bone, ligaments and muscles). The more collagen you have, the more likely you are to have stronger ligaments and muscles, which could reduce the risk of tears and injury.

Some people may be more predisposed to injury than others. 'Running is beneficial for most people but there are some individuals that may get injured more often or develop arthritic changes quicker than others,' says Mailer. 'There are many factors that affect our joint health, such as genetics, body weight, strength levels, volume of exercise and how we run.'

Losing even a small amount of weight will help protect your joints. When you consider that up to three times your bodyweight goes through the joints when you run, losing just 2 lbs can reduce stress on the knees by up to 6 lbs.

Good leg strength is also important. 'If you don't have good strength in the lower limbs then you may be putting too much stress on your knees, ankles or spine,' says Mailer.

'This is extremely important, as the stronger you are in your quadriceps (front thighs), hamstrings (rear thighs) and glutes (bottom), then the more protection your joints will have.'

Overall, the long-term benefits of running will stand you in good stead. Let's refer back to Professor James Fries from Stanford University's study that lasted more than 20 years. With participants now in their 70s and older, the study has shown that runners have stayed fitter than non-runners and running is not associated with greater risk of joint disease. The team from Stanford University found that adults who run consistently could expect to have 25 per cent less musculoskeletal pain and less arthritis than non-runners when they get older. It also showed that runners have a lower risk of osteoarthritis and hip replacements.

IS IT WORTH TAKING A JOINT-CARE SUPPLEMENT WHEN RUNNING REGULARLY?

There has been conflicting evidence regarding the benefits of joint supplements such as glucosamine, chondroitin sulphate and cod liver oil with patients suffering from osteoarthritis and for joint health in general. (Glucosamine and chondroitin sulphate are natural substances found in the cells of cartilage.) Many clinical studies have demonstrated that supplements such as glucosamine can help in a reduction in symptoms and pain with people suffering from osteoarthritis, but it has also been seen that many subjects failed to respond to treatment.

However, they are not deemed to be harmful, so it's up to you whether or not you decide to take them.

WHAT'S THE BEST SURFACE TO RUN ON?

The best surfaces to run on in terms of cushioning are flat grass (as long as it's not too hard) and the treadmill (which has some cushioning) rather than tarmac or concrete. Most people think that trail running (off-road running) can be a good option to reduce impact. This can be true but it depends on how challenging the terrain is. Very uneven, soft or muddy trails can put added pressure on the knee joints, as the knees try to stabilise your body and keep you upright while you cover uneven surfaces.

'Running on tarmac or pavements is generally going to cause more wear and tear on a joint than running on a softer grass surface,' says physiotherapist Mark Buckingham. 'However, all of those surfaces come with their own issues. Grass surfaces like bowling greens can be ideal, but most off-road running is not that flat. It's going to have ruts, it's going to have rabbit holes.'

Some road surfaces can be challenging, too. 'Road surfaces are not necessarily flat and smooth,' adds Buckingham. 'You've got undulation, cambers, potholes and kerbs.'

It's worth varying your routes as much as possible. If you always run the same route, in the same direction, you could be putting strain on one side of the body, such as the knee or hip, especially if your route has cambered pavements. From time to time, change or reverse the route.

While running downhill may feel easier, there is more impact through the knee joints. Your body is trying to slow you down and decelerate the momentum of gravity pulling you down.

AM I TOO OLD TO START RUNNING?

No one is too old to run unless they have any major health or mobility issues. But it's a common misconception that older people can't run. Bupa commissioned a survey of 2,055 adults in March 2014 and found that 93 per cent of those aged 50 to 65 didn't run. The study also uncovered that, even among regular runners, 60 per cent of those taking part in the survey claimed that once they are over 50, they won't be able to run.

If you are older or have health issues but want to start running, make sure you get the go-ahead from your GP first, especially if you've been sedentary for some time.

TV presenter and former royal correspondent Jennie Bond took up running at the age of 63. She successfully completed the Bupa London 10,000 run (6.25 miles) in May 2014. Other examples of older runners include Ron Hill, now aged 77, who, at the time of writing, has run every day since 1964, and Fauja Singh, who started running at the age of 81 and has completed multiple marathons. He retired from marathon running in 2013 at the age of 102 (yes, you read that correctly!).

CAN I RUN WITH HIGH BLOOD PRESSURE?

When you are first diagnosed, it may take some time to get your blood pressure stable and to a safe level for exercising. But once it's controlled then it's safe and beneficial for you to run, as regular cardiovascular exercise may help lower your blood pressure in the long term. However, it's important to start slowly and build up gradually. Run at a moderate intensity when you first start, which means you shouldn't be gasping for breath and should be able to have a brief conversation with the person next to you. Listen to your body. Stop if you feel light-headed, dizzy or unwell, and visit your GP if this happens.

DO I NEED TO RUN REGULARLY TO IMPROVE HEART HEALTH?

Yes. But from your very first session, however slow you run, you will have made a positive change to your heart muscle. To maintain that change you need to go again, ideally three times per week. Within a few weeks your heart health will have improved significantly.

WILL DISTANCE RUNNING DAMAGE MY HEART?

Running will strengthen your heart, by decreasing your resting heart rate and improving the size and strength of the heart itself. Longer, slower runs will improve the endurance of the heart muscle, working it steadily at a moderate heart rate. Doing faster, shorter blasts will improve the strength and power of the muscle. A combination of both is ideal to improve your overall fitness.

There is some evidence to suggest that, during very long runs, such as marathons or ultramarathons (ultramarathons being any distance over 26.2 miles), temporary damage can occur. Studies in both high-level athletes and recreational marathon runners have shown that there are changes to the heart muscle function and signs of damage that develop during the 26.2 miles. Experts don't yet fully understand the significance of these changes and what they mean to long-term heart health. They do, however, seem to be transient and resolve in the majority of people after a few weeks of recovery. A study of recreational marathoners found that the changes were more severe in those that had the lowest fitness levels and had done the least training. This means that proper marathon training is essential.

CAN RUNNING CAUSE STRESS INCONTINENCE?

Running won't directly cause stress incontinence (where urine leaks involuntarily when you run) but if your pelvic floor muscles are weak then you may suffer from leakage. Women's pelvic floor muscles can be weakened by childbirth but it's also a common problem for middle-aged women who haven't had children (and is thought to affect around 30 per cent of women who exercise). It only affects a small proportion of men. If you are having leaks when you run, visit your GP. Exercises to strengthen your pelvic floor muscles will usually help and your GP will be able to advise you.

IS TREADMILL RUNNING AS EFFECTIVE AS RUNNING OUTSIDE?

It depends what you want to achieve. If you simply want to start running and build a good base of fitness, the treadmill could be a good place to start, as you can stop when you want to and it's also easier to time harder intervals with periods of recovery. Running outside is generally harder because you will encounter varied terrain as well as the elements. The only variables on the treadmill are the speed and incline, which you can change depending on how hard you want to work. If used effectively, the treadmill can be a good way to get fit and burn calories.

However, if you are training for a race that has lots of uneven, muddy terrain, or steep hills, you'll need to experience these conditions during your training.

CAN I RUN IF I'M PREGNANT?

Medical experts will advise against taking it up if you've never done it before. If you're already an experienced runner, you may want to run up to a certain point in your pregnancy, before switching to lower impact exercises like cycling, rowing or using the cross-trainer.

During the first trimester, you don't want to get too hot. Keeping your body at a normal temperature is important for healthy formation of cells in the developing baby. Therefore, wear layers that can be easily removed and wear a well-fitting sports bra. Start doing pelvic floor exercises to prevent leaks.

During the second trimester, start to take it easy. By the third trimester – or even earlier if you begin to find running uncomfortable – you may want to switch to low-impact cardiovascular exercise.

On a general note, a hormone called relaxin (present in the body when you are pregnant) will reduce joint stability, which can increase injury risk, so don't overdo it and make sure you have good footwear (see chapter 3).

CAN I RUN EVERY DAY?

It's generally not advisable, as your body needs time to recover. For most people simply looking to get fit, lose some weight and improve their health, running three to four times per week – with a day of rest or low-impact cardiovascular exercise in between runs – is ideal. If you do run more frequently, have a day of complete rest at least once a week. If you're doing a lot of running, do plenty of stretching (see p.50).

I HAVE ASTHMA. CAN I STILL RUN?

It's important to visit your GP or asthma nurse first and get the green light to exercise before you start running. If your asthma is well controlled – which means you rarely experience any symptoms – then it should be OK to run if you start slowly and gradually (and it certainly hasn't stopped Paula Radcliffe). Make sure you have your reliever inhaler (which is usually blue) on you at all times so that if you do experience any symptoms you can deal with it quickly. If you have been prescribed a preventer inhaler, take it every day (usually morning and evening). Remember it's normal for your heart to beat faster and your breathing to increase, and you may feel a bit out of breath when you first start. However, if you start experiencing asthma symptoms, like coughing or wheezing, feeling very out of breath, you have a tight chest or start gasping for air, then stop or slow down. If your inhaler doesn't relieve the symptoms, then stop altogether. You will then need to visit your GP for further advice.

Asthma UK, the UK's leading asthma charity, has highlighted that regular cardiovascular exercise, like running, should actually improve your lung function and help you manage your asthma symptoms. Running also helps you lose weight, which could reduce your symptoms and lower your risk of having an asthma attack. (Visit www.asthma.org.uk for more information.)

IS IT TRUE THAT WOMEN ARE MORE PRONE TO KNEE INJURIES THAN MEN?

In theory, yes, and it comes down to physiological differences. The female pelvis is wider, so the angle of the thighbone to the lower leg bone is greater in women than men (called the 'Q-angle'). This can increase stress at the knee joint and the kneecap. The female knee is also smaller and there is a smaller space for the deep cruciate ligaments to move in the knee, meaning they can be torn or more easily irritated. However, having good balance, strong glute (bottom) muscles, core and thigh muscles can all help reduce the risk of knee injuries.

WILL RUNNING MAKE MY NIPPLES BLEED?

If you're a male doing a long run like a half-marathon or a marathon, it is possible that the rubbing of your T-shirt against your nipples might cause some chafing or minor bleeding. You can cover your nipples with plasters, but they do have a tendency to come off. Applying Vaseline may be a better solution. This is generally not a problem during shorter distances.

WILL RUNNING CAUSE UNCOMFORTABLE CHAFING?

If you're doing long distances, you may get some chafing of the inner thighs or nether regions, but the sensible solution is to generously apply Vaseline to prevent sensitive skin rubbing. For most people doing recreational running and moderate distances, it's less likely to happen. If you are carrying some excess weight then you may get a bit of chafing between the inner thighs and under your arms during distance running. Before longer runs, also apply Vaseline on the soles of your feet, on the heels and in between the toes, on the nipples and, for males, on the genitals.

WILL MY TOENAILS FALL OFF?

Again this is usually linked with long distances, but it can happen if your running shoes are too tight and your toes are rubbing against the ends of your shoes, causing repeated trauma to the nail. When the black nail is bruised and becomes separated from the nail bed, eventually it will fall off. Buying at least one shoe size larger should help avoid the problem.

AT A GLANCE

- You don't have to be thin to run
- Loading of the joints can improve joint health
- Older runners stay fitter in later life than non-runners
- Flat grass and the treadmill provide some cushioning
- You're never too old to start running if you're healthy
- The treadmill could be a good choice for new runners
- You can run with asthma if it is under control

" I enjoy running with friends but essentially I like to get lost in my thoughts and run on my own. "

RHALOU ALLERHAND, FREELANCE
JOURNALIST, DISTANCE RUNNER

CHAPTER 3

GET THE RIGHT KIT FIRST

Before you start running, there are two key things to do. Firstly, it's worth visiting your GP and getting the go-ahead to run, especially if you've been sedentary for a long time. The next task is to get the right kit.

Let's start with your feet. You'll need the right pair of running shoes for your foot type. It's well worth visiting a specialist running store rather than a general high street sports shop. Good stores include Runners Need, Sweatshop, and Run and Become. If you visit a general sports store, the staff won't necessarily have any knowledge of running shoes, and you'll most likely end up choosing a pair that you like the look of, which may not suit your running style. If you choose the wrong shoes, it could cause an injury as your mileage increases, because the shoes won't necessarily offer the right support.

GOOD KNOWLEDGE

Those who work in specialist running shops are usually runners themselves and will have a good knowledge of different shoe types. They will typically ask you how much mileage you intend to do every week. They may ask you to run briefly on a treadmill or outside the store (for a minute or two) so that they can check your running gait (how you run) or they may ask you to run on a floor tile that takes an imprint of your foot and reveals how your foot strikes the ground.

Most importantly, they will recommend the right type of shoe for your foot strike and whether or not your feet pronate.

WHAT IS PRONATION?

Pronation is normal during running. As the heel strikes the ground, the inside of the arch drops downwards. 'It's normal for the foot to do this to help to absorb force from the ground,' says physiotherapist Tim Allardyce. 'However, some runners suffer with overpronation, that is the inside arch of the foot drops inwards too far.'

Running shoes are designed to counter the effects of pronation. Too much pronation can cause injuries like shin splints, hip pain, back pain and even groin strain. 'The arch of your foot is designed to help absorb and dissipate much of the force from the ground when you run,' says Allardyce. 'If that arch is completely lost (due to the rolling in of the foot), your foot does not absorb so much and the force goes into the shin, knee and hip. Second, the knee turns inwards, which places uneven stress going into the shin, knee and hip joint.'

Some of us pronate more than others. Broadly speaking, there are several different types of pronation:

- Underpronation – also known as 'supination'. This is when the foot doesn't pronate much at all, meaning the foot doesn't roll inwards and the outer side of the foot hits the ground, so that the impact goes through the lower leg. Common injuries can include stress fractures and shin splints as well as increased pressure on the ankles, shins and hips. *Best shoe type: cushioned shoes.*
- Neutral or normal pronation – the foot rolls inwards to up to 15 degrees and makes a stable platform on the ground. There is minimal inward roll and the foot comes in complete contact with the ground. This is a fairly efficient stride and the force of the impact is distributed quite evenly. A neutral runner is generally less

likely to get injured as the body is generally happier in a neutral position. *Best shoe type: neutral shoes.*

- Overpronation – this is when the foot moves more than 15 degrees inwards when it hits the ground. The ankle rolls to the inside and the big toe is forced to work hard to push the foot off the ground again. Injuries that can be caused by overpronation include shin splints, *Plantar fasciitis* (also known as jogger's heel) and Achilles tendonitis, as well as bunions. *Best shoe type: maximum support or structured cushioned shoes.*

- Severe overpronation – when the foot rolls excessively inwards in the late stage of the running gait. This can mean a large amount of weight is transferred to the inside of the foot. The more you pronate, the greater the risk of injury. *Best shoe type: maximum support.*

WHAT ABOUT BAREFOOT AND MINIMALIST SHOES?

You may have read the media hype about 'barefoot' or 'minimalist' shoes and wondered if they are worth trying. Barefoot shoes are very light and small, and offer a limited amount of protection. This is intentional as they are designed to simulate the feeling of running barefoot, as our ancestors did thousands of years ago. They have attracted a lot of interest, but are not suitable for everyone. It's important to consider how different our environment is from that of our ancestors. Tim Elsey, assistant manager of Runners Need in London's Liverpool Street, says: 'Look at what the very best athletes do. They never train in barefoot shoes and only step down to minimal or racing shoes when they do sessions or races. We live in a world that is by and large entirely unnatural. Nowhere in nature will you find complete uniformity of the surface we tread on in our roads. When we repeatedly strike a perfectly hard and flat surface, our bodies go through the same movements stride after stride. There is no break or respite until we head off-road.'

While barefoot shoes may be suitable for short distances on grass to wake up and switch on the muscles of the feet, they aren't necessarily ideal for distance running on roads and other hard surfaces.

Minimalist shoes offer more cushioning than barefoot shoes but are lighter than normal cushioned or stability running shoes. They have less material in them and are often slightly less durable than a normal cushioned shoe. They are designed to encourage runners to adopt more of a mid-foot or forefoot running strike, rather than a heel strike. (Some experts believe that when you heel strike, you are creating a braking effect, which puts more force through the joints.)

'Minimalist shoes have a flatter profile to the ground, are lighter in construction and allow more natural flexion of the foot,' says Elsey. Some converts to minimalist shoes will argue that by providing more contact with the ground, they provide more feedback through the foot. In theory, this would help make the muscles in the foot stronger.

Cushioned shoes offer more protection and are heavier. 'Cushioned shoes have more substance under the sole,' adds Elsey. 'They are stiffer and have a steeper drop from heel to forefoot, which facilitates a heel strike.'

Lighter runners can get away with less cushioning than heavier runners, but if you are intending to run longer distances, you would most likely benefit from a cushioned shoe for the bulk of your training, especially if you are running on roads.

BUYING YOUR FIRST RUNNING SHOES

Some people will naturally need more cushioning and support in their trainers than others, especially those who are carrying more weight, have flat feet or those who are naturally heavier through their feet. Flat-footed runners will have less shock absorption in their feet, as the arches are designed to absorb shock. Someone with flat feet may therefore be better suited to a cushioned shoe.

Jonanthan Quint, EMEA marketing manager for leading running brand Saucony, says: 'Starting with a good standard pair of running shoes (for example, cushioned) is a good place to start – to dive straight in with minimalism could give you more to consider when you've got enough to consider already.'

Quint adds: 'Minimalism is great for people who are looking to maybe make a few changes to their running style, to get on to the toes, and run slow and lighter, but to start with, I would go for comfort. Go and have your gait checked and take the advice of a specialist store.'

This is good advice as shoe type is a complex subject. You could talk to different runners about shoes and they may give you differing opinions based on their own personal experiences.

It's best to try on several pairs of shoes recommended by your local running store and go with the pair that feels the most comfortable. 'I would be led by the advice you get in store as to the direction to go in,' says Quint. 'Also make sure that what you put on your feet is comfortable, as otherwise you won't want to wear them.'

If you are aiming to run longer distances like a half-marathon or marathon, then go for a more cushioned shoe. You may hear runners talk about the 'drop' of a shoe – this simply means the difference in the height of the shoe between the heel and forefoot. Minimalist shoes tend to have a 4-mm drop, while more cushioned shoes will have a thicker heel – either an 8-mm or 12-mm drop – to provide more cushioning. Shoes with a higher drop will help you strike the ground with your heel, while shoes with a lower drop will encourage more of a mid- or fore-foot strike.

Running coach Nick Anderson from RunningWithUs (www.runningwithus.com), who has more than 20 years' experience of coaching Olympians and recreational runners, says: 'Heavier people should definitely run in more cushioned shoes.'

GO FOR COMFORT

Choosing the right shoe can be confusing but, in the end, it comes down to what you feel comfortable wearing. You'll need to go up a shoe size or even a size and a half bigger than your normal shoe size, as your feet swell when you get hot.

If you intend to run off-road on muddy, uneven trails, then you'll need a pair of trail shoes, which have better grip on the soles to prevent you slipping in mud. They will also be firmer, but with enough flexibility to cope with uneven surfaces. Many are also lightweight and water repellent. Your local running store can advise you more on the best trail shoe for your foot type.

WHEN TO CHANGE YOUR SHOES

Running shoes typically last for around 300 to 500 miles, depending on your running technique. There are also some visible signs that your shoes may be worn out. 'Turn the shoe over and push your thumbs into the ball of the sole and see how much flex you get back,' says Jonathan Quint from Saucony. 'The shoe is not built to flex in that direction, so if it does and doesn't fight against you then that's a key sign that the midsole is wearing out. Creasing in the midsole (the layer of white spongy material between the outsole and upper part of the shoe) and wear on the outsole would mean the shoes are really worn out, as the outsole is typically made of carbon rubber and is a stronger material, so shouldn't be wearing out.'

FOOT PROTECTION

It's also worth investing in a pair of running socks that are twin-skinned and that wick the sweat away from the feet, which will reduce the risk of blisters. Running socks usually offer a better fit and reduce sweat build-up. They can also regulate the temperature of your feet, as they are made from polyester and nylon.

When trying on running shoes, wear the socks you will run in so that you know the shoes fit well.

TECHNICAL KIT

If you don't want to spend too much money on running clothing when you first start out, you could run in light tracksuit bottoms and a T-shirt in moderate weather conditions. However, as the weather becomes more extreme and you begin to increase mileage, you'll be grateful for some technical running kit. A pair of running tights or capris and a top that wicks sweat and moisture away from the body will make you feel more comfortable. Cotton jogging bottoms may feel comfortable during normal weather but on a wet day they will feel heavy.

Some running fabrics contain sun protection factor (SPF) in them – most brands include a sticker on the item telling you the level of sun protection offered – which is ideal for running on hot days. Technical running kit is made from lighter materials so that heat can escape from the body, as well as having wicking properties, to help wet kit dry quickly.

During cold weather, layers are ideal. A base layer will keep the heat in, so adding a light wicking top over it and a light jacket is perfect. When you've warmed up, you can pull your jacket sleeves up or remove light layers and tie them around your waist.

Buy a cap to keep the rain out of your eyes and a beanie to keep your head warm during cold weather. Running gloves are also worth buying to keep your hands and especially your fingertips warm when running in the cold, as it's not practical to try and run with your hands in your pockets!

SUPPORT YOUR ASSETS

An essential item of kit for women is a supportive sports bra designed for running (even if you have a small bust). There are different levels of impact, and you'll need a high-impact level bra. Breasts are supported by delicate structures called Cooper's ligaments. These ligaments are inelastic, meaning once they've been stretched, due to lack of support, they won't return to their normal pre-run state. A two-year study of 70 women at the University of Portsmouth found that not only do breasts bounce up and down when we run, they also move from side to side in a figure of eight motion.

When it comes to buying a sports bra for running, there are two types to choose from – compression and encapsulation. Compression bras flatten the breasts to the chest wall. Encapsulation bras have moulded cups that hold each breast separately and allow them to move independently. Racerback bras spread the weight more easily and wider straps improve weight distribution.

When choosing a sports bra, bear in mind your ribcage contracts and expands when you run to allow for greater oxygen demand, so you may need a bigger bra than your normal size. Your bra should not show any cleavage or your breasts won't be fully supported. The bra should be a snug fit with no gapes or bulges.

Good brands include Shock Absorber, Sportjock, Berlei, Lynx Sportswear, Panache, Moving Comfort and Anita. Repeated washing will reduce the support and elasticity of your bra, so you'll need to change it every six to nine months (depending on how often you run) or approximately every 40 washes.

AT A GLANCE

- Visit a specialist running store when buying shoes
- Buy at least a size bigger than your normal shoe size
- Cushioned shoes are generally better for beginners and running longer distances
- Buy a pair of trail shoes if you are running off-road
- Change your running shoes every 300 to 500 miles
- Buy running socks to avoid blisters
- Invest in technical running kit

" If you can walk, you can run.
You are never too slow, old, big,
or uncoordinated to run. "

KATHRINE SWITZER, BEST-SELLING AUTHOR
OF *MARATHON WOMAN*, RUNNER OF
39 MARATHONS, THE FIRST WOMAN TO
OFFICIALLY RUN THE BOSTON MARATHON
IN 1967 AND FORMER WINNER OF
THE NEW YORK CITY MARATHON

Chapter 4

IT STARTS WITH YOUR HEAD

Anyone can run. Provided you're healthy, you're good to go, even if you're not exactly in peak physical condition. It doesn't matter how old you are, what size you are or when you last exercised – if you're mobile, you can run. It's really that simple. It may be a bit challenging at first but you will be surprised at how quickly your stamina will improve if you do it regularly. It's important to start sensibly, which means getting your pace right from the beginning. If you begin at a moderate pace, you will improve your stamina quite quickly. It's best to do the first few runs on your own, so you won't feel any pressure to keep up with someone else and you can set your own pace.

BRINGING THE FAMILY TOGETHER

Harriet Sakon from Alberta, Canada, began running in 2003 at the age of 42. 'I started running because as I was pushing my double stroller with my little ones in it, and they were yelling, "Go, Mummy, faster, faster!", I ran a block and nearly collapsed, and my children looked very disappointed in their pathetic little ride.

'I joined a "Learn to Run" class and I found that I enjoyed the camaraderie of the other runners. I joined the 10-km class, then the half-marathon class. Finally, I joined the full-marathon class and for my first marathon, I ran the full, and my husband and sister-in-laws all ran the relay. As a family, we completed it together. The best thing about running is how it pulls families and friends together.'

If you doubt your ability to run, imagine how many countless other people felt the same way at first. There are numerous examples of people who have transformed their health, fitness and quality of life through running. Overweight people have slimmed down and reduced their risk of obesity and diabetes. People in their seventies and eighties can still run marathons. If you look at the start line of the Virgin Money London Marathon, you'll see that running doesn't discriminate. All shapes and sizes line up to run 26.2 miles. Appearances can be deceiving. A fit runner is hard to define purely by body shape alone. You'll see runners in heavy rhino costumes overtaking runners in normal running kit. You'll see larger people overtaking slimmer people. You'll see older folk overtaking youngsters. Don't be so quick to judge on appearances. Don't be too quick to judge yourself. You *can* do it and you don't have to be slim, fit or young to try.

Most of the conversations I've had with people who think they 'can't run' will lead to a recollection of a bad experience. They tried it before and found it hard, so they gave up.

Think about what happened to give you a negative view of your running ability. When you tried it in the past, did you set off too fast? Were you forced to run by your PE teacher at school and were criticised for not being quick enough, or for wanting to stop?

You're in control now, so your experience will be different this time. You can choose how far or how long you run. Let past experiences go. Running can be a bit challenging at first, but it will soon get easier. It's simply about finding the right pace and having adequate rest periods.

It doesn't matter how short or slow that first run is – start running and do it regularly. Don't give up after that first run. Remember the famous quote from Henry Ford: 'Whether you think you can, or think you can't, you're right.' Don't let yourself choose to fail.

Look for success stories to get you inspired. Here are a few examples:

PATIENCE PAYS OFF

Mel Abrams, mother and former headteacher, has completed half-marathons, a marathon and even an Ironman event (which comprises a 2.4-mile swim, a 112-mile bike ride and a 26.2-mile run – all in one day). Now clearly very fit, Mel recalls how tough it was when she first started. 'I was proud of doing about half a mile at first,' she recalls. 'Then I entered a 5-km Race for Life at Hyde Park and found it really, really hard. It seemed so long. But when it finished I was totally high on adrenaline and hooked.'

For Mel, running was a challenge to overcome with patience and persistence. 'It was a challenge because I was a bit overweight and unfit but I still enjoyed it,' she recalls. 'I could feel myself getting stronger and more able to keep going.' Her advice for new runners is quite simple: 'Stop sprinting,' she says. 'You'll get too exhausted, injured and demoralised. Run easy until it's getting hard, and then walk for a couple of minutes. Repeat a few times. Then go home, drink, eat and rest. Then do it again and keep doing it. Believe in yourself. Everyone can run – we just do it at different paces and speeds.'

Cardiac rehab specialist nurse Lorraine Voisey, from Leicester, started running when she was nearly 50 years old and weighed 16 stone. She admits she found those first few runs 'extremely tough', but again, persistence paid off. 'I really wanted to get healthy, not have high blood pressure and set an example to my boy,' Lorraine recalls. 'I definitely didn't enjoy it for the first few weeks. I really didn't think my body could cope with it or ever get the "Runner's High" I kept reading about.'

Lorraine persevered, and went on to lose 5 stone and also completed the London Marathon, which, funnily enough, gave her a real high at the end. She adds: 'Being a runner really makes you feel invincible.'

LIFESTYLE CHANGE

Owen Sawford, from Buckinghamshire, began running in 2009 as an ex-smoker who wanted to get fit. 'As strange as it sounds, I finished smoking and I saw running as the perfect suppressant to pushing away any urge to visit the dark side again!' he recalls. 'The first few weeks of running I found tough but I soon enjoyed it. At the end of the day, the race is only ever with yourself.'

Owen went on to run the London Marathon in 2014, raising money for charity, and losing 2 stone. He insists: 'Anyone can run. Humans are built for running after all! I would say to any new runner to take it easy and pace yourself. Within a few weeks, you'll get quicker.'

If you are serious about wanting to improve your health, look slimmer and have more confidence, then it's worth persisting. It will get easier.

FIND A ROLE MODEL

Finding a role model is a good way to build your confidence. There must be someone you know who has transformed their life through running or exercise. Maybe it's someone who has surprised you by what they have achieved. People can achieve incredible things, even when the odds are against them.

Dave Wise, a sports and travel writer from Kent, is one of the most inspirational runners you could hope to meet and is lucky to be alive. 'In 2006 I was offered a press trip to run the Colombo Marathon in Sri Lanka,' he recalls. 'I'd never run a race of any kind before, but I thought you can't write about anything unless you've experienced it, so I decided to try to run it.

'A few weeks after training began I was attacked by a gang of English football fans. They gave me a ruptured spleen, broken ribs and a one in four chance of living. I had three weeks in hospital and couldn't leave the house for many months afterwards. The doctors had left my spleen to heal on its own but said it might burst if I had any contact at all, like brushing up alongside somebody in the street. I was a mental wreck. The Colombo Marathon organisers invited me again to run it, two years after their first invite, and training for it gave me something to focus on.'

Dave slowly began to get fitter and went on to take part in the marathon he'd signed up for two years earlier. 'Finishing that race was a sort of beginning for me, putting the past behind me and starting afresh. It was a very slow run, and a very hot one. After I'd run about 25 km [about 15 miles], I was ready to stop, I was so exhausted and in great pain all over, especially my stomach. A bus pulled up in front of me, black exhaust smoke was everywhere, a cow wandered into my path and a three-wheeled taxi nearly hit me, all in the space of a few seconds. I sat down and felt really sorry for myself. *Why me?* I thought. *Why did I get attacked?* And then I looked up, and saw on the other side of the street, through all the traffic, a man with no legs, and he was pulling himself along the street with his arms. And then I thought, *Why not me? I don't deserve any special treatment, why shouldn't I have some hardship in my life?* And so I got up and walked and ran, then walked again, and finished the race.

Since then I've run 42 marathons, lost about 3 stone and gone vegan. The spleen still bothers me now and again, but only if I really overdo it.'

Dave's story proves that you don't need to be fit to start running. He had suffered a huge ordeal that had not only threatened his health but also his life. Yet he didn't let it hold him back.

POSITIVE THINKING

Others have faced similar hardships and even tragedy. Liz Goodchild used running to help her cope with bereavement by signing up for the Royal Parks Ultra, a 31-mile race, after losing her mother. 'My mum was very depressed and took her own life,' she says. 'I decided that I wanted to do something positive in her memory, so I worked with Mind to raise awareness. When the training got hard, I thought about all the people who had sponsored me.'

'Those first few runs felt awful,' adds Liz. 'I honestly felt like I was going to pass out. Everything hurt. My legs, my lungs, my feet, and I only managed to run for about 100 metres! But something inside me knew it was a good thing to do. Running helped me in so many ways. It made me realise that I was capable of so much more, physically and mentally. From hardly being able to run 100 metres to running hilly ultramarathons, I started to question what else I could be achieving and began to set goals, not just in running, but in life as a whole.'

Liz completed the ultra-race and has since retrained as a life coach, inspiring others to achieve their goals. She adds: 'I have such a better understanding of who I am because of running. I've developed a strong mindset and no longer settle for a "treading water" type of life. If you get into the habit of thinking you can't do things you want to do, you won't ever do those things. Everyone started as a beginner. Build up slowly. I think there's something deeply holistic about running. It's what our bodies were designed to do.'

AT A GLANCE

- Anyone can run
- Running will get easier quickly
- It's never too late to start running
- Self-belief is crucial
- Put past experiences aside
- Find role models for inspiration
- Our bodies were built for running

" I could feel myself getting stronger
and also more able to keep going. "

**MEL ABRAMS, OFFICE WORKER, RUNNER
AND IRONMAN COMPETITOR**

Chapter 5

HOW TO START RUNNING

Before you start, it's worth giving some thought to where you'd like to run. Consider what type of environment would best suit you. Do you like green space? If yes, then the local park might be perfect. If you think you'd prefer running indoors at first, then the treadmill at your local gym could be a good starting point. Just make sure it's a location where you feel safe and comfortable. Some people hate polluted main roads or busy urban locations, where you have to dodge pedestrians. Others dislike the uneven terrain of running on trails. Some like the predictable nature of the treadmill (you have total control over speed and incline), while others find it boring and prefer varied scenery. If you're not a treadmill fan, but you're not sure how far you'll be able to go, then a short loop around the block is a good way to start.

ESSENTIAL ITEMS

It's always worth carrying a mobile phone, some cash and, if it's a hot day and you're trying out a new route, some water. It's also worth carrying some identification. Add your partner's or a friend's mobile number to your phone under the name of 'ICE', which stands for 'in case of emergency'. Hopefully it won't ever be needed, but it offers peace of mind.

Before you start your first run, it's important to get your body ready for the exercise you're about to do. A warm-up gradually raises the heart rate, preparing it for activity and also gets the joints ready. When you warm up, the joints will release a fluid called synovial fluid, which effectively lubricates the joints, getting them ready for exercise.

Before you start the warm-up, begin with some dynamic stretches (stretching with movement), which can include the following:

- For quadriceps (front thighs): knee bends – stand with good posture, bring one leg behind you as if you were trying to kick yourself on the bottom. Repeat on the other leg.
- For hamstrings (rear thighs): stand with one foot about a stride length in front while you push the hip of the back leg forward, stretching the front of the hip. Repeat on the other leg.
- For glutes (bottom): stand with good posture and, keeping your torso upright, swing one leg backwards and forwards, making sure the movement is only coming from the leg. Repeat on the other leg.
- For calves: find a step or kerb near a wall and rest against it for balance, if required. Then, standing upright, gently place one foot on the edge of the step, letting the heel drop backwards, and rise upwards on to your toes. Repeat on the other leg.

Perform four to five repetitions of each on both legs. Always do this before a run.

MAIN WARM-UP

Start with a slow walk, picking up the pace and progressing into a brisk walk for the first 5 minutes. (As you get fitter, you'd want to progress into a light jog and then a gentle run.) Make sure you spend at least 5 minutes warming up. You should feel warm before you start running.

COOLING DOWN

When coming to a finish, gradually reduce your pace down from a run or a jog into a slow walk, rather than just stopping.

STRETCH OUT

Always stretch the quadriceps, hamstrings, glutes and hip flexors, back, shoulders, chest and triceps. Hold each stretch for at least 30 seconds. You can find demonstrations of all of these stretches at www.chrismacfitness.com.

STARTING OUT

The best way to start as a brand new runner is to jog for 30 seconds to 1 minute, then walk for 1 to 2 minutes and repeat this in intervals up to four times.

Your very first run would typically look like this:

Dynamic stretches

Warm-up:
5 minutes of walking (starting slowly and
gradually increasing into brisk walking)

Main session:
Jog for 30 seconds to 1 minute
Walk for 1 or 2 minutes
Repeat x 4

Cool-down:
4–5 minutes of gradually reducing
speed to a slow walk

Post-run stretch (see 'Stretch out', p.51)

BUILD IT UP GRADUALLY

Experiment with the walk/run intervals based on how you feel. If the running interval feels easy, then jog for 1 minute and walk for 1 minute, then repeat based on the previous example. Increasing either the running intervals or reducing the walking intervals will make the session harder.

Each week, try to make small increases in the amount of time you run or reduce the walking intervals.

If you want to build up to running 5 km (3.12 miles), following a training plan is a good way to improve your stamina gradually. Over the page is an example that you can follow strictly or use as a rough guide. The plan demonstrates how to steadily increase volume, and how to schedule a typical training week so that you give your body adequate time to recover in between runs.

	Monday	Tuesday	Wednesday
Week one	Run 1 min/walk 2 mins x 5 = 15 mins	Rest	Run 1 min/walk 1 min x 5 = 10 mins
Week two	Run 1 min/walk 2 mins x 6 = 18 mins	Rest	Run 2 mins/walk 1 min x 6 = 18 mins
Week three	Run 2 mins/walk 2 mins x 6 = 24 mins	Rest	Run 3 mins/walk 1 min x 4 =16 mins
Week four	Run 3 mins/walk 2 mins x 4 = 20 mins	Rest	Run 4 mins/walk 2 mins x 4 = 24 mins
Week five	Run 5 mins/walk 2 mins x 3 = 21 mins	Rest	Run 5 mins/walk 1 min x 5 = 25 mins
Week six	Run 6 mins/walk 1 min x 4 = 28 mins	Rest	Run 9 mins/walk 3 mins at brisk pace x 3 = 36 mins
Week seven	Run 7 mins/walk 1 min x 3 = 24 mins	Rest	Run 12 mins/walk 3 mins at brisk pace x 2 = 30 mins
Week eight	Run 8 mins/walk 1 min x 4 = 36 mins	Rest	Run 15 mins easy pace/ walk 3 mins at brisk pace then run 5–10 mins easy pace at the end = 23–28 mins

Thursday	Friday	Saturday	Sunday
Rest/stretch	Rest or gentle cross-trainer or cycling or swimming 15 mins	Run/walk 15 mins with as few walk breaks as possible	Rest, yoga class or gentle stretching
Rest/stretch	Rest or gentle cross-trainer or cycling or swimming 20 mins	Run/walk 20 mins with as few walk breaks as possible	Rest, yoga class or gentle stretching
Rest/stretch	Rest or gentle cross-trainer or cycling or swimming 22 mins	Run/walk 25 mins with as few walk breaks as possible	Rest, yoga class or gentle stretching
Rest/stretch	Rest or gentle cross-trainer or cycling or swimming 25 mins	Run/walk 30 mins with as few walk breaks as possible	Rest, yoga class or gentle stretching
Rest/stretch	Rest or gentle cross-trainer or cycling or swimming 25 mins	Run/walk 35 mins with as few walk breaks as possible	Rest, yoga class or gentle stretching
Rest/stretch	Rest or gentle cross-trainer or cycling or swimming 30 mins	Run/walk 37 mins with as few walk breaks as possible	Rest, yoga class or gentle stretching
Rest/stretch	Rest or gentle cross-trainer or cycling or swimming 35 mins	Run/walk 40 mins with as few walk breaks as possible	Rest, yoga class or gentle stretching
Rest/stretch	Rest or gentle cross-trainer or cycling or swimming 40 mins	Run/walk 45 mins with as few walk breaks as possible	Rest, yoga class or gentle stretching

SETTING THE RIGHT PACE

Many people set off too quickly and run like they're sprinting for the bus. Use the 'talk test' to tell whether or not you're running at the right speed. This means running at a pace that would allow you to talk (speaking entire sentences) if you had someone next to you. If they were to ask you a question, you'd be able to answer. You know you're going too fast if you can barely speak or only utter one word.

You can also use a tool called the Rate of Perceived Exertion (below), which grades your intensity level (how hard your run feels) on a scale of one to ten. Ten is that feeling of sprinting – which you don't want. You want to run at an intensity level of between four and six.

10	Maximum effort – sprinting for a bus or train you desperately want to catch
9	Very hard – difficult to maintain this pace
7–8	Vigorous activity – borderline uncomfortable and short of breath – can't speak much at all
4–6	Moderate activity – breathing heavily but can hold a short conversation
2–3	Light activity – feels like you can keep going for hours – easy to breathe and talk
1	Very light activity – hardly doing anything at all

It may take time to find the right pace for you but experiment and see how you feel. Slow down when you need to, increase the rest periods if need be and don't push yourself too hard during those early runs. The aim is to build up a positive association with running.

WHY COOL DOWN?

At the end of your run, slow down gradually, rather than just stopping suddenly, as the latter can cause dizziness or even fainting. The legs have more blood moving through them during exercise and suddenly stopping can mean blood pools in the lower body. Gradually reducing speed also gives the muscles a chance to lengthen out, and allows your heart rate and breathing to return to normal gradually.

AFTER YOUR RUN

When you get home, drink water, eat a healthy meal or snack containing carbohydrates and protein (see chapter 8) and reflect on your run. Keep a running journal for motivation. Write down what you did and how you felt physically and mentally. When you look back on it in a few months' time, you'll be amazed by the progress you've made.

THE FOLLOWING DAY

Have a rest the following day or do some low-impact exercise like walking, cycling, swimming or using the cross-trainer. Do some light stretching. Rest days are an important part of the recovery process. A weekly yoga class is also recommended to give you a thoroughly good stretch.

PLAN AHEAD

It's best to get into a routine and plan when you'll be running: three times a week is ideal. A good example of a weekly running schedule would be to run on Monday, Wednesday and Friday, or Tuesday, Thursday and Saturday. You can do low-impact exercise on non-running days, though I'd recommend one day of complete rest each week.

PEAKS AND TROUGHS

Some days you will naturally have more energy than you do on others. Your ability to run well on a given day depends on many variables, such as:

- How much sleep you've had
- The quality of your sleep
- How much water you've had to drink
- How much you've eaten during the day
- What you've eaten during the day
- Whether you've had any alcohol the night before
- Your stress levels in general
- The time of day you run (early risers will prefer morning runs, while night owls will feel stronger in the evenings)

CONSISTENCY IS KEY

During the first month, try to be consistent with your routine. Get into a habit of running at a certain time. If you're feeling tired or stressed, run anyway. The chances are, your fatigue is more mental than physical and the run will actually make you feel better.

If you can run consistently, without missing a week, your stamina will improve quickly.

Each week, you can increase time or volume, but make sure it's not by more than 10 per cent in total. So if you run for a total of 45 minutes in week one (say three lots of 15 minutes), make sure you don't run for more than a total of 50 minutes in week two. Gradually build volume. Then on week five, pick the volume back up again and you'll feel fresh and raring to go.

AT A GLANCE

- Choose your preferred environment before you run
- Carry a mobile phone, cash and, on a hot day, water
- Carry some identification with you
- Perform dynamic stretches and warm up before your main session
- Alternate between walking and jogging/running
- Always cool down and stretch at the end
- Find the right pace for you – don't worry if it seems slow
- Track your progress for motivation
- Rest or do light low-impact exercise the following day

" Running has not only got me fit but also boosted my confidence and self-esteem, making me more assertive in many other areas of life. It has also given me a more positive outlook in general. "

EVA HATFIELD, ACCOUNTANT,
MARATHON RUNNER

Chapter 6

TRAIN SMART

Once you become more confident in your ability to run, you may want to run more often or increase your distance. This is all positive, but be careful – injuries can strike even the most experienced runner. You may be overdoing it if you are:

- Increasing mileage or time too quickly
- Running every day and not giving your body a chance to recover
- Trying to get faster and achieve a 'personal best' on every run
- Making every run a hard session (a harder run should always be followed by a rest day or an easy recovery run)
- Trying to keep up with other runners who may be faster than you

TRY DIFFERENT RUNS

As you start to see signs of progress, it's easy to overdo things. Keep having the rest days you need and increase volume gradually. Listen to your body. If you feel tired, go for an easier run.

Vary the types of running you do to improve your fitness and prevent you from doing endless long runs that can lead to repetitive type of injuries. Different types of running sessions include the following:

- Long, slow distance
- Threshold
- Out-and-back run
- Intervals
- Fartlek
- Hill training

Long, slow distance runs

These are sessions performed at a comfortable intensity, which means at a pace that allows you to continue for long periods of time. Think of someone training for a marathon doing a long run. They will need to keep going for several hours.

Threshold runs

This is where you have blocks of time where you push yourself to the edge of your comfort zone. On the RPE (Rate of Perceived Exertion) scale, you would be working at around an eight out of ten during a threshold run. You might do blocks of threshold for 3 to 4 minutes and then recover by running at a moderate pace for 2 minutes, then repeat this a further three to four times. As you get fitter you would look to increase the duration of the harder periods. As you're running faster than normal, a threshold run will boost your fitness which means you should find it easier to run at your normal speed. This type of run is quite strenuous and is only recommended when you become fitter and more experienced.

Out-and-back runs

Ideal if time is tight. It means running to a certain point in, say, 15 minutes, then turning around and heading back home, with the aim to get home in less time, for example, in 14 or 13 minutes. The challenge element of the 'back' part of the run will keep you motivated to push a bit harder than usual.

Interval runs

You would typically run at a challenging pace for a fixed period of time (1 or 2 minutes, for example), then slow down and run at a moderate pace to recover (for the same amount of time) and then repeat this, say, four times. Intervals will increase your fitness and are an effective way to burn more calories and increase your metabolic rate. The treadmill is perfect for doing intervals, as it times the intervals for you, but they can also be timed outside with a stopwatch. Again, interval sessions with high intensities is only recommended for experienced runners.

Fartlek training

'Fartlek' translates as 'speed play' and it means quite simply running at random bursts of speed. After warming up, you might sprint for 10 seconds, jog for 30 seconds, turn and change direction and sprint again, then run at a reasonable pace, change direction again, and so on. It's unplanned. Fartlek training is commonly used for sportspeople, like footballers, who have to adapt to sudden changes in pace and direction during a game. It's less relevant for recreational runners unless you take part in team sports, though some runners find it useful for getting fitter for a sprint finish at the end of a race. Again it's not generally recommended for beginners.

Hill training

This simply means factoring in some hills when training. Find a route that contains hills, or you can add more structure to your training and find a specific hill, then run up it, jog down gently to recover and then repeat several times. This is tough but ideal if you're training for a race that is likely to be hilly.

RECOVERY TIME IS ESSENTIAL

To avoid injuries, you shouldn't do intervals more than once or twice per week and not on two consecutive days, as you need to allow the body time to recover. The same goes for threshold runs and hills. Equally, you wouldn't do two long runs back to back, as the high volume could lead to a greater injury risk. Once a week is ideal for all of these sessions. You'd follow a hard session like intervals or threshold with a rest day or a gentle recovery run the next day.

BUY A FOAM ROLLER

Legs feeling stiff? A foam roller is a tube that can massage out knots in the muscles. You simply roll it over tight muscles, such as quadriceps, hamstrings or calves, and by applying pressure, the foam roller can help break up those knots. Also known as myofascial release, it is similar to a deep-tissue sports massage. For anyone who runs regularly, it's a must-have piece of kit. They aren't expensive and you can buy them from most sports shops and online. Many gyms also have them available for use.

VARY YOUR RUNS TO GET FITTER

Many people building up their mileage can fall into the trap of clocking up too many long runs in one week. Simply adding volume and doing more can increase injury risk. Even if you're training for a half-marathon or a marathon, you only need to do one long run of more than 90 minutes per week. The more you run, the more important regular stretching becomes.

AT A GLANCE

- Follow a harder run with a gentle recovery run or rest the next day
- Use the foam roller to massage out tight knots in the muscles
- Listen to your body – if your muscles ache then take a day off
- Vary the type of runs you do to improve your fitness

" The body is an engine. It only runs well on the right fuel. I've learned the hard way that the wrong fuel can leave you lacking in energy, drive and well short of your destination. "

EDDIE MACDONALD, PHOTOGRAPHER, RECREATIONAL RUNNER

Chapter 7

COMMON RUNNING INJURIES

When running begins to feel easier, you'll start to enjoy it, and you'll rely on it to reduce stress and unwind. So you can imagine how frustrating it feels if injury strikes. But some injuries could be avoided as they can sometimes occur when minor aches and pains are ignored, or when we run too much. If something hurts, you should see a physiotherapist straight away and always follow their advice, even if it means not running for a while.

If you get injured, it's crucial to listen to your body and give yourself adequate time to recover. A key way to help reduce the risk of injury is to try low-impact cross-training, to give your body a break from running. Examples include swimming, cycling, rowing or using the cross-trainer. It can also include classes that raise the heart rate and work the cardiovascular system. Group indoor cycling (also known as 'spin'), where you cycle to motivational pumping music (with hills, sprint intervals and easier periods of recovery) is a good way to exercise the heart and lungs. Low-impact cross-training will help you keep fit and reduce injury risk because there is minimal impact on joints.

LOOK AFTER YOUR JOINTS

Strength training (training with weights or doing body weight-resistance exercises like squats or lunges) can help reduce injury risk, specifically joint problems. When we run and land on the leg, the quadriceps (front thighs) take up to 60 per cent of the impact of the ground away from the knee, so if they are weaker, then we will increase load on the knee joint and this could contribute to injury.

Here are some common running injuries. But don't be discouraged from running – just be sensible. Lots of the injuries here are caused by overdoing it or poor biomechanics (bad running style). If you train wisely (see chapter 6), you'll hopefully be able to avoid them. We have explained how to treat them in this chapter, but if the pain or injury persists, then visit your GP or a physiotherapist.

PLANTAR FASCIITIS (ALSO KNOWN AS JOGGER'S HEEL)

What is it? A condition that involves pain at the heel, most commonly on the inside. It is related to the structure called the plantar fascia, a band of thick fibrous tissue that comes from the heel bone and stretches under the foot and up to the toes. *Plantar fasciitis* is thought to be due to overuse and microtrauma to the tissue, which then leads to pain. Contributing factors can be tight calf muscles or foot muscles, change of footwear and running too much, too soon.

Solution: rest and don't run. Stretch the calf muscles and the foot to help reduce tissue tightness. Applying ice or using a foam roller on the sole of the foot can also help.

ACHILLES TENDONITIS

What is it? There are many different injuries that can occur near and to the Achilles tendon – which is the strongest and thickest tendon in the human body, originating in the middle of the calf and connecting the calf muscles to the heel bone. Two of the most common disorders are Achilles tendonitis and Achilles tendinosis. Achilles tendonitis is an acute inflammation (rapid and short-lived) of the Achilles tendon, while Achilles tendinosis is a long-lasting chronic degenerative disorder of the tendon.

In Achilles tendonitis, overuse is the main cause, where too much load is placed through the tendon and micro-tears of the tendon occur, causing inflammation.

Solution: rest, ice, stretching and a gradual increase in strength. Strength can be increased by doing body-weight double-leg heel raises (two sets of ten to 15 repetitions per day, then adding five to ten repetitions each week). As strength improves, you would progress to single-leg heel raises, again doing two sets of ten to 15 repetitions. This should completely resolve the problem, with the tendon repairing and recovering fully. However, sometimes with too much overloading, the tendon does not repair and the tendon structure becomes disrupted without inflammation. The changes in the tendon will then give a longer period of pain and can be more difficult to treat. Approaches to treating Achilles tendinosis include rest, ice and stretching.

ITB SYNDROME

What is it? A common injury in running that occurs on the outer side of the knee. The ITB, or iliotibial band, is a long, thick piece of connective tissue on the outside of the leg extending from the outside of the pelvis, over the hip and knee, and inserting just below the knee.

It is believed that ITB syndrome is caused by friction over the outer part of the knee, such as a bursa (fluid-filled sac) or by compression in the underlying fat tissue, causing pain and swelling.

Solution: rest, applying ice regularly and stretching. A foam roller can also help in reducing tightness by gently rolling over the middle part of the ITB, i.e. the middle part of the outer leg above the knee and below the hip. Strengthening the glute muscles can help. Other treatments such as massage and acupuncture have been known to also help recovery.

SHIN SPLINTS

What is it? Shin splints is the name given to pain at the front of the shin that occurs during exercise, like running, and can relate to many injuries such as a stress fracture or, most commonly, medial tibial stress syndrome (MTSS). MTSS is thought to be caused by pulling and traction to the outer layer of tissue covering the bone called the periosteum, located by the deep calf muscles. It seems that MTSS is associated with quickly increasing exercise intensity or duration of training, uneven surfaces, and excessive pronation and muscle weakness.

Solution: treatment first involves ice and rest. Applying ice to the shin for approximately 10 minutes for the first three days can help reduce pain. Resting and offloading the leg by not walking for long periods and avoiding walking uphill will help allow the tissue to recover. Once pain has subsided and walking is comfortable, it is important to make a gradual return to running. It's worth visiting a physiotherapist or podiatrist as you may have weakness of the lower leg muscles. They can advise you on how to return to running safely and also how to strengthen any weaknesses in the legs that may have caused the injury.

IS IT SHIN SPLINTS OR A STRESS FRACTURE?

Many people wonder what the difference is between shin splints and a stress fracture. Shin splints is a generic term for shin pain, while a stress fracture is a specific injury or diagnosis. A stress fracture is an incomplete or partial fracture that has been caused by too much stress and loading on a local area of bone over a period of time that can be confirmed with an X-ray. This is most common in the foot and shinbone with runners.

WHAT IS 'RUNNER'S KNEE'?

Runner's knee is a generic term for pain at the front of the knee relating to the patella (kneecap). The pain is usually from overloading the patella due to poor biomechanics (bad running style) or muscular imbalances. For example, when we bend and straighten our knee, the patella moves in a groove called the trochlea, which is known as 'patella tracking'. If our quadriceps (front thigh) muscles are too weak or the ITB is too tight, this can disrupt the tracking of the patella, therefore causing pain. There are other biomechanical factors that can contribute, such as poor single leg stability. We see this when landing on one leg and the knee rolls inwards, which then causes the patella to track outwards. This would then overload the patella and, over time, start to cause discomfort or pain.

Solution: by maintaining good quadriceps and hamstring (rear thighs) strength, as well as good flexibility of our calf muscles, ITB and quadriceps, and having good single leg stability (see p.99), we can reduce the chance of suffering from runner's knee.

AT A GLANCE

- Always see a physiotherapist if pain strikes
- Listen to your body and rest when you need to
- Remember your physiotherapist knows best – don't return to running too soon
- Cross-training can help keep you fit while your body recovers

> **"** I'm a busy working mum with a hectic life and going out for a run gives me a chance to enjoy 'me time', with no other distractions, no background noise – just me doing something positive for my health. I love it. **"**

GERI GORNELL, RECEPTIONIST, RECREATIONAL RUNNER

CHAPTER 8

NUTRITION FOR RUNNING

One of the benefits of taking up running is that you'll naturally want to pay more attention to what you eat – or, to be more specific, the *quality* of your nutrition. You'll want to eat healthier foods so that you feel good while you run and have the energy to keep going.

Knowing what to eat can be confusing as there are so many conflicting opinions, as well as various diets that are way beyond the scope of this book. Nutrition is a controversial topic. Some runners will tell you to eat more carbohydrates. Others will say they run well on a lower carbohydrate diet and more protein. One thing we do know is that carbohydrates and stored fat will provide the energy you need for running, while protein will help aid recovery post-run – and carbohydrate stores should be replenished after a run.

It's worth experimenting with different healthy foods to find out what works best for you. Keep a food diary to see how your food and drink consumption affects your energy levels during a run.

Avoid very low-calorie diets, even if you are running for weight loss (see chapter 9). Not only is it difficult to have a decent run on very limited calorie intake, but such diets can be detrimental to your health as you may be missing out on essential vitamins and minerals. (For optimum health, nutritional experts recommend that we eat a wide variety of foods.)

If you feel bloated or experience abdominal discomfort during a run, cut back on high-fibre foods, such as beans, nuts and pulses, but don't cut them out completely, as they are nutritious – just make sure that your last meal before a run isn't too high in fibre.

Consider the timing of when you eat and whether or not your portion is too large before a run. What might be perfect for one runner might cause tummy troubles for another. It's the same with energy gels and drinks. Some runners can tolerate most gels and drinks, while others are more sensitive and need to make more careful choices.

ENERGY FOR RUNNING

In an effort to try to simplify what is clearly a complex subject, during exercise, our bodies obtain energy from three main sources: carbohydrates, fats and protein. Energy needs vary between individuals and also depend on our age, weight, muscle mass, gender and how active we are. However, the average daily calorie requirements are 2,000 for women and 2,500 for men. (These are the recommendations of the UK's Department of Health Guidelines as published by the Food Standards Agency.) The recommended daily intake for each are as follows:

- Carbohydrate: 50–60 per cent of your total calorie intake
- Fat: 25–30 per cent of your total calorie intake
- Protein:10–15 per cent of your total calorie intake

Carbohydrates

Carbohydrates are the body's preferred source of energy. There are two types of carbohydrate – simple and complex. Simple carbohydrates include foods like honey, sweets and refined products, such as cakes, biscuits, white bread, white rice, fruit juice and dried fruit. They provide an instant release of energy, as they are quickly absorbed into the bloodstream.

Complex carbohydrates

These have a higher nutrient density than simple carbohydrates. Examples include wholegrain cereals, pasta, porridge, and vegetables, such as lentils, peas and beans, as well as starchy vegetables, like sweet potatoes, carrots and parsnips. Complex carbohydrates provide a slow release of energy, so eating a meal with complex carbohydrates 2 to 4 hours before a run should provide you with sufficient energy. However, if you are doing a longer run of more than 90 minutes, you may need additional simple carbohydrates during your run that are swiftly absorbed into the bloodstream and therefore provide energy immediately. Energy gels and energy drinks are good examples of simple carbohydrates. If you are doing shorter distances that are less than 90 minutes, you won't need to take gels or energy drinks while running.

Fat

Fat is the body's second preferred source of energy during exercise. Fat is energy dense (it contains 9 calories per gram, compared with carbohydrate and protein, which each contain 4 calories per gram) and is the body's largest store of energy.

When you have depleted your carbohydrate stores (after around 90 minutes of continuous running), your body will turn to fat stores for more energy.

Protein

Protein is the third and least preferred source of energy by the body. However, it plays a key role in recovery after exercise, as it helps repair damage to muscle fibres that occurs during exercise. Good protein sources post-run include eggs, milk, lean meats, poultry and fish. According to the American College of Sports Medicine, if you're regularly active, you'll need to consume around 1.2–1.5 g of protein per kilogram of body weight each day to get a sufficient intake. So if you weigh 70 kg (approx. 11 stone) for example, you'd need at least 84 g of protein daily. As a rough guideline, a protein bar will typically contain around 20 g of protein, an egg (including yolk) will have around 6 g of protein (depending on the size), a 100 g chicken breast will have around 31 g of protein and a cooked salmon fillet weighing 100 g will have around 25 g of protein.

Try to avoid empty calories

Chocolate, crisps, cakes, biscuits and alcohol don't offer any nutritional benefits. The only exception here is dark chocolate, which contains antioxidants. However, it should still only be eaten occasionally, as it's high in calories and sugar.

Got milk?

Chocolate milk has been noted for its recovery benefits after exercise, according to a study published in *International*

Journal of Sport Nutrition and Exercise Metabolism. When you compare it with plain milk, water or sports drinks, it has double the carbohydrate and protein content.

Carbohydrate intake

The question of whether to increase your carbohydrate intake as a runner can be a difficult one as there are many variables. 'It depends on your current intake, and whether you are looking to lose or maintain weight, and, again, activity level and intensity,' says nutritional therapist Sarah Ellis.

It comes back to the quality of your food. The best carbohydrates for runners include non-processed wholegrains, such as brown rice, fresh fruits, vegetables and legumes. If you are aiming to lose weight, wild rice, sweet potatoes and vegetable carbohydrate sources are lower in calories and provide more nutrients than white rice, pasta or bread.

EATING FOR EFFICIENCY

When it comes to fuelling morning runs, good breakfast choices include porridge with berries and semi-skimmed milk, scrambled eggs on wholemeal bread, or a healthy smoothie. If you run early before work and you don't feel like eating anything, you should have the energy for a run as long as you ate a healthy meal the night before. If you feel like you need a small snack, a banana will do the trick.

After your run

Post-run, it's best to eat within half an hour if you can (regardless of what time of day it is). 'Protein is needed after exercise to aid recovery,' says Ellis. 'Carbohydrates also need to be eaten after exercise to replenish glycogen stores. If you want to lose weight, opt for low-calorie, dense foods to fill you up and help you avoid overeating. Lentil soups, leafy greens and hard vegetables, such as carrots and broccoli, will make you feel full and give you energy.'

The overall message here is to experiment with different foods and try to avoid empty calories that don't provide any nutritional benefits. 'It's trial and error for most people,' says Ellis. 'There is no "one size fits all" diet for everyone.'

Some foods are reported to help reduce inflammation in muscles after a run. 'Have some antioxidant-rich fruits – such as berries – and vegetables after exercise to reduce muscle soreness,' says nutritionist Christine Bailey. 'A snack 30 to 45 minutes post-exercise and then a normal meal later would be fine.'

Importance of fluids

As well as your post-run snack, consuming fluids after your run is also important. 'For longer runs you may be looking at around 24 oz of fluid for every pound lost during a run, 12–15 g of protein and 35–50 g of carbohydrate immediately after a run,' says Christine Bailey. 'If you're not hungry, a 12-oz glass of low-fat chocolate milk, or a protein fruit smoothie, half a cup of trail mix of roasted nuts and seeds with dried fruit, and a cereal or sports bar with enough carbohydrates and protein (but under 200 calories) should work fine.'

On a more general note, here are some easy ways to improve your diet and help provide the energy you need for your running:

- Eat five portions of vegetables per day – they are nutrient-rich and low in fat and calories. Adding vegetables to soups is an easy way of increasing vegetable intake.

- Drink more water – most of us need at least eight glasses daily, but you'll need more if you exercise (see 'How much water and when?' box on the next page).

- Cut back on alcohol – the occasional tipple is fine, but remember it's full of sugar and empty calories.

- Eat a nutritious snack at least an hour before you run, or eat a small meal 2 to 4 hours before a run – good options for pre-run meals include a chicken sandwich, jacket potato with beans or tuna, tuna salad with rice, or porridge.

- Eat lean protein – chicken and fish are better choices than red meat, which is high in saturated fat. Too much saturated fat can cause inflammation.

- Eat omega-3 fats – these are natural anti-inflammatory foods and the best sources include oily fish, such as sardines, mackerel, trout and salmon (three portions a week is ideal), or flaxseed oil (2 tablespoons per day), chia seeds or walnuts.

- Cut back on refined foods, such as white bread, rice and pasta, and swap them for wholegrain rice, oats and quinoa. These will help stabilise your blood sugar levels and avoid energy dips.

WHY DRINK WATER?

Water is essential as it transports nutrients to various organs, regulates your temperature and circulation, and also plays a role in maintaining your energy levels. Even if you are just doing a steady run, the quality of your run will be affected by dehydration. Losing just 2 to 3 per cent of your body weight in fluid can lead to impaired performance. A 4 per cent loss of your body weight in fluid can lead to a decrease in endurance, meaning you won't be able to run for as long.

The exact daily intake you need depends on the weather (you'll need to drink more on hot days), the intensity of your run and how hydrated you were to begin with. It's important to drink the recommended daily amount of around 3–3.5 litres if you're a male and 2–2.5 litres if you're a female. Try to drink water throughout the day gradually rather than all in one go and remember if you're feeling thirsty, you're already dehydrated.

HOW MUCH WATER AND WHEN?

Before your run: drink about half a litre up to 2 hours beforehand, then drink around 200 ml around 5 minutes before you run.

During your run: sip water every 10 to 15 minutes if you are running for more than an hour.

After your run: drink more water – if you want to be precise, weigh yourself before and after your run. This will help you determine how much sweat you've lost. For every half a kilogram you lose, replace it with two cups of water.

REPLACING LOST ELECTROLYTES

If you have sweated a lot and have only consumed water during a long run of more than 90 minutes, you need to replace lost salts to rebalance your electrolyte levels in the body. Electrolytes are minerals found in blood and cells, and are essential to activity as they regulate bodily fluids, helping support muscle and nerve function. Sodium, potassium, magnesium and calcium are the four major electrolytes that maintain the body's fluid balance.

If electrolyte levels are low after a long run, your muscles may feel weak. 'If you have ever cramped up after a long run, gone for a run on a hot summer's day or you tend to sweat a lot, the chances are you will need electrolytes,' says Christine Bailey. 'Keeping your electrolytes balanced is key for successful training and optimum performance. If your electrolytes are imbalanced, you may experience muscle fatigue or cramping.'

More worryingly, the long-term effects of not replacing lost electrolytes can include kidney failure and seizures. 'Urine colour is one of the easiest ways to assess your hydration and electrolyte levels,' adds Christine. 'Ideally it should be pale straw in colour.'

If you have completed a long run of 90 minutes or more, an electrolyte sports drink is a good idea, as these are formulated to replace lost salts in the body – good brands include High5, SiS and Torq. High5 and Torq both offer electrolyte tablets that dissolve in water and are fruit-flavoured, making them palatable. Avoid electrolyte drinks that contain high amounts of simple sugars or artificial sweeteners – powdered sachets and tablets are often the best option. Simple sugars are fructose, glucose and sucrose, and artificial sweeteners include aspartame, saccharin and sucralose.

AT A GLANCE

- Carbohydrate is the body's preferred energy source. It can fuel around 90 minutes of continuous exercise (around 2,000 calories within the body)
- Try to improve the quality of your diet
- Find the eating plan that works for you
- Avoid very low-calorie diets
- Try to eat non-processed wholegrains
- Eat a meal 2 to 4 hours before you run
- If you miss a meal, eat a small snack 1 hour before you run
- Eat as soon as possible after your run, consuming carbohydrates and protein
- Consume a sports drink if you run for more than 90 minutes to rebalance fluid levels in the body

" Before you reach for that chocolate bar, ask yourself... is 30 seconds of pleasure worth 2 hours of guilt? "

MARK HATFIELD, NUFFIELD HEALTH
FITNESS ACADEMY TRAINER,
OBSTACLE RACE COMPETITOR

Chapter 9

RUNNING FOR WEIGHT LOSS

People run for different reasons. Some people run so that they can eat what they want, some run to lose weight, while others run to improve their health or reduce stress levels. However, weight loss is often a key reason why many people start running in the first place. Running burns a lot of calories compared with other forms of exercise like walking, gentle cycling and swimming – in fact, it burns an average of 100 calories per mile. But to lose weight, it must be combined with a healthy eating plan. If you run two to three times a week and overeat, you won't lose weight. You might even gain a few pounds.

Even marathon runners can gain weight during training, usually because they believe: 'I'm doing a marathon so I can eat what I want.' Yet it's virtually impossible to burn off the calories if you are eating too much. You'd literally have to do hours and hours of running. If the average chocolate bar contains around 300 calories, you'd need to run approximately 3 miles or for around 30 minutes to burn it off. A Classic American Hot pizza from a well-known chain of pizza restaurants in the UK contains 807 calories. You'd need to run at least 8 miles to burn off the calories.

In the end it comes down to controlling calories and expending more energy (calories) than you consume, as well as making good-quality food choices. Reduce calorie intake sensibly, choose healthy foods and the pounds will gradually fall off. One pound per week is a sensible rate of weight loss. You would need to create a weekly calorie deficit of 3,500, or a daily calorie deficit of 500 calories, to achieve this goal.

CALORIE GUIDELINES

The approximate guidelines for daily calorie intake are 2,000 calories for women and 2,500 for men. However, these are only guidelines and if you want to be more precise about your calorific needs then your age, weight and activity levels should be taken into consideration. To work out roughly what you need, multiply your weight in kilograms by 25 (it is assumed that the average person uses 25 calories of energy at rest per kg of bodyweight) to get your resting metabolic rate (your body burns calories at rest simply to keep functioning). If you are sedentary (you do little or no exercise), multiply your resting metabolic rate by 20 per cent to get your total daily calorie allowance. If you're moderately active, multiply your resting metabolic rate by around 50 per cent. Examples are below:

For a 60 kg female who is moderately active:
60 x 25 = 1,500 calories needed for RMR (resting metabolic rate) x 50 per cent = daily calorie needs of 2,250

For a 70 kg male who is moderately active:
70 x 25 = 1,750 calories needed for RMR x 50 per cent = daily calorie needs of 2,625

The real skill lies in being honest and working out how 'active' you are, and this can be difficult. A sedentary person is someone who doesn't take part in regular sport or exercise and spends a lot of time sitting at a desk or watching television. The activity you do is part of your daily routine and is low intensity, meaning you can breathe normally.

A moderately active person is someone who exercises but gets less than two and a half hours per week of moderate intensity aerobic activity (exercise where you breathe harder but can hold a conversation, such as a light jog).

Someone with high levels of activity would typically exercise regularly at least three times a week doing exercise like running, where your heart rate increases substantially, or comparable physical activity, where your breathing rate increases and the exercise is vigorous. You might spend 2 to 3 hours per week in total exercising.

The key is not to go below your resting metabolic rate, as this is not only dangerous to your health (leading to a reduced immune system and lower energy levels), but it can also lead to muscle wastage. Remember, your body has two preferred energy sources during exercise: carbohydrate and fat. If the body doesn't have sufficient stores of either, because you are not consuming enough calories, it will reluctantly convert protein into energy. Protein is not a preferred source of energy and it also means your body is eating into lean muscle tissue. Since most people would want to lose fat, rather than lean muscle tissue, this is clearly counter-productive. Your body will also hold on to calories consumed if you're limiting your intake too much. It knows that food is scarce, so it cleverly tries to conserve energy.

If you are unsure how to estimate your daily calorie needs, there are some good online tools that can help. Perhaps the most respected among nutrition experts is the Harris–Benedict Equation – a method used to calculate your basic calorie requirements before you add on additional calories based on activity levels.

SNACK IN MODERATION

Don't go for long periods of time without eating anything, or you'll be ravenous at the end of a run and will be more likely to overeat. Be careful with snacking, too. Nutritionist Christine Bailey normally only recommends snacking if you really need to, as not snacking too often helps give your digestion a rest and also helps maintain better blood sugar levels (which can prevent cravings that can lead to overeating).

Thirst can often be confused with hunger. If you feel hungry, drink a large glass of water and wait for 20 minutes. You may find the hunger goes away.

We've talked a lot about calorie intake, but it's important to consider healthy food choices. Nutritionists are keen to point out that not all calories are created equally. Bailey says: 'Different calorie sources can have vastly different effects on hunger, hormones, energy expenditure and the brain regions that control food intake. Even though calories are important, in many cases, simple changes in food selection can lead to the same, or better results, than calorie restriction.'

GOOD CHOICES

Eat wholemeal carbohydrates such as brown rice, brown bread, wholegrain pasta and lean protein (such as fish or chicken without the skin on). For weight loss, you will need to watch your carbohydrate intake even if you are running. If you are worried about whether you'll have enough energy to run when cutting carbohydrates, remember that you can still get carbohydrates from vegetables and fruit. Eat plenty of fresh fruit and vegetables to make you feel full. Make snacks small and limited to healthy choices like a small handful of nuts, fruit or oatcakes.

RUNNING TO BURN FAT

Now let's look at your running sessions. Here are some ways to plan your weekly running schedule to boost weight loss:

- Run regularly – you need to run frequently enough to burn off sufficient calories – aim to run three to four times per week and do low-impact cardio (cross-trainer, rower or a spin class) on two other non-running days, so that you exercise a total of five to six days per week. (Be careful not to overdo it though. You should only do this amount of exercise if you have built up your fitness levels. Always stop and rest if you feel any pain or discomfort during exercise.)
- Add high intensity intervals once a week – interval runs are considered more effective for weight loss than low- or moderate-intensity cardiovascular sessions as they burn more calories in less time, making them easier to fit into your schedule. A study published in the *Journal of Physiology* found that about 20 minutes of high-intensity interval training provided the same benefits as longer exercise sessions that focused on endurance work.

High intensity intervals are also thought to create a metabolic effect where your body continues to burn more calories after exercise. A study presented by Florida State University in 2007 reported that subjects who did high-intensity cardiovascular training burned almost 10 per cent more calories 24 hours after exercise than those doing lower-intensity cardiovascular exercise for longer.

To structure an interval session, run hard for 1 or 2 minutes (at around 7–8 out of 10 on the RPE scale) and then run at a moderate pace (around 5–6 out of 10 on the RPE scale) to recover for 1 minute or 2, then repeat. This will also improve your fitness, allowing you to run for longer during steady runs, increasing total calorie burn throughout the week.

Add a threshold run once a week – this means running just on the edge of discomfort for fixed periods time – such as 3 minutes at a faster pace (at around 8–8.5 out of 10 on the RPE scale), followed by 2 minutes of recovery, repeated for a total of three to four blocks.

Add hill-training sessions to your weekly running schedule – hills are more challenging than running on a flat surface, so you'll burn more calories doing it. As a general guide, you can expect to burn 10 per cent more calories for each degree of incline. So if you are running at a 5 per cent incline, you will burn 50 per cent more calories than running on a flat surface. Make sure the hill isn't too steep – a gradient of 6 to 10 per cent will be fine. You can also use the treadmill for hill training.

Add one long, steady run per week – this is to increase weekly calorie burn overall – but increase duration gradually. Add 10 per cent to your total weekly volume and no more. As a rough guide, if you run for an hour you would burn around 600 calories, depending on age, weight and speed.

- Vary your running sessions – your body will quickly adapt if you only do the same run and pace each time and it will begin to feel easy. If you only ever run on a flat surface, going off-road and doing some trail runs from time to time will increase exercise intensity (and therefore calorie burn) as you will have to work harder to tackle uneven surfaces.

- Use an app to track calories burned and calories consumed – it's easy to eat more than you realise and it's also easy to overestimate calories burned. MyFitnessPal enables you to log every activity and meal, and counts calories for you. It'll also give calories burned during exercise. Active Goals is another useful app that enables you to set your own goals for each run, be it by time, distance or calories burned. RunKeeper is a free app that records distance and calories burned.

WHAT ABOUT THE 'FAT-BURNING ZONE'?

Some people believe that moderate-intensity cardio will burn more fat than shorter, more intense sessions, because at lower exercise intensities you are supposed to be working in the 'fat-burning zone'. The theory is that you're using stored fat for energy, instead of carbohydrates. There is some truth in this but it's not anywhere near as effective as it sounds.

Low-intensity exercise, like walking or jogging slowly, will access fat stores for energy, whereas high-intensity exercise, like interval training, will access more stored carbohydrates. When you work harder, your body will typically use carbohydrates as well as stored fat for energy.

But in order to work at a lower intensity, you'll be jogging at a slower speed. This means you'll burn fewer calories in total. If you walk for 20 minutes and burn 100 calories, this is clearly not going to be as effective as running for 20 minutes and burning 200 calories.

Remember: it's calories in vs calories out for weight loss – you need to expend more calories than you consume.

While you need to train frequently enough and hard enough on some sessions, it's also easy to overtrain. You need to find a balance between working hard and not overdoing it. If you've never done hill sessions or interval runs before, don't suddenly introduce them into your weekly training routine all at once, or you could risk injury. Build fitness gradually, and then add in harder sessions. If you're new to running, you'll probably lose weight anyway, as you'll be increasing calorie burn overall.

AT A GLANCE

- Run frequently throughout the week
- Use interval and threshold sessions to burn more calories
- Add in cross-training sessions to increase total calorie burn
- Hill sessions burn more calories than running on flat surfaces
- The fat burning zone isn't as effective as it sounds

" I've found that most things that are good for you, that propel you way out of your comfort zone, are challenging. Running has now taught me to build my 'emotional' muscles – to push against resistance. I've developed a strong mindset. "

LIZ GOODCHILD, LIFE COACH

Chapter 10

BUILDING STAMINA AND IMPROVING YOUR RUNNING

You've made it this far. You're hooked on running. You enjoy it and you can already feel yourself getting fitter. You want to improve and increase your mileage. So how can you train to improve without training like an elite athlete?

Building stamina is partly a case of 'time on your feet' – which means increasing your running volume – and also making sure you have adequate rest days to let your body recover, as well as doing strength training to support your muscles during running. Don't increase weekly volume too quickly – do it gradually. Follow the 10 per cent rule.

Hill training and threshold runs will increase fitness. If you can cope with hard hills, you will find flat surfaces much easier by comparison. Threshold runs will push you out of your comfort zone, meaning your normal running speed will get easier.

FROM 5 KM TO 10 KM

If you're comfortably running 5 km and you want to increase your distance to 10 km, then you could follow this training plan. The plan assumes that you're already running a 5-km distance and can make the leap from 5 km to 10 km of continuous running, but it's still OK to take occasional walking breaks.

If you are using this training plan for a 10-km race, you will need to add an additional two weeks at the end for you to taper, which means gradually reducing the amount of time you'd run in the last fortnight, so that your body is fresh for the start line. You'd have an extra rest day in the last two weeks, then reduce the time of your long run down to approximately 40 minutes in week nine and 30 minutes in week ten. You would also have complete rest two days before the race.

BOOSTING SPEED

What if you want to get faster? A simple tip is to run with someone slightly faster than you. This will naturally inspire you to run at a pace that pushes you slightly out of your comfort zone. It's also worth joining a running club. Most running clubs have groups for improvers. To find your nearest group, visit www.runengland.org.

If you want to get faster over shorter distances, try the following:

Up to two interval-training sessions per week – 1 minute hard, 1 minute easy or 2 minutes hard, 2 minutes easy (repeat a total of four to five times) to improve your aerobic fitness (keep the work/rest ratios the same but experiment with the length of the intervals) or try a weekly threshold session – as shown on the next page. Don't do this on consecutive days. Allow the body time to recover.

	Monday	Tuesday	Wednesday
Week one	Rest and stretch	Threshold run 4 mins harder, 2 mins easy x 3 = 18 mins	Gentle cross-trainer or cycling (or other low-impact exercise, e.g. rowing, swimming) = 30 mins
Week two	Rest and stretch	Threshold run 4 mins harder, 2 mins easy x 3 = 18 mins	Gentle cross-trainer or cycling (or other low-impact exercise, e.g rowing, swimming) = 30 mins
Week three	Rest and stretch	Threshold run 4 mins harder, 2 mins easy x 3 = 18 mins	Gentle cross-trainer or cycling (or other low-impact exercise, e.g rowing, swimming) = 35 mins
Week four	Rest and stretch	Threshold run 4 mins harder, 2 mins easy x 4 = 24 mins	Gentle cross-trainer or cycling (or other low-impact exercise, e.g rowing, swimming) = 35 mins
Week five	Rest and stretch	Threshold run 4 mins harder, 2 mins easy x 4 = 24 mins	Gentle cross-trainer or cycling (or other low-impact exercise, e.g rowing, swimming) = 40 mins
Week six	Rest and stretch	Threshold run 5 mins harder, 2 mins easy x 4 = 28 mins	Gentle cross-trainer or cycling (or other low-impact exercise, e.g rowing, swimming) = 40 mins
Week seven	Rest and stretch	Threshold run 6 mins harder, 2 mins easy x 3 = 24 mins	Gentle cross-trainer or cycling (or other low-impact exercise, e.g rowing, swimming) = 45 mins
Week eight	Rest and stretch	Threshold run 8 mins harder, 2 mins easy x 3 = 30 mins	Gentle cross-trainer or cycling (or other low-impact exercise, e.g rowing, swimming) = 45 mins

On week five, the long run has deliberately been reduced down to 45 minutes (from 55 minutes the previous week) to give your body an easier week and allow for some recovery. The distance goes up to 60 minutes in week six.

Thursday	Friday	Saturday	Sunday
Hill training 20 mins (run up, jog down to recover)	Strength training (see p.99 for ideas) and stretch	Rest or yoga	Run 40 mins at a moderate intensity (with as few walk breaks as possible)
Hill training 20 mins (run up, jog down to recover)	Strength training and stretch	Rest or yoga	Run 45 mins (with as few walk breaks as possible)
Hill training 25 mins (run up, jog down to recover)	Strength training and stretch	Rest or yoga	Run 50 mins (with as few walk breaks as possible)
Hill training 25 mins (run up, jog down to recover)	Strength training and stretch	Rest or yoga	Run 55 mins (with as few walk breaks as possible)
Hill training 25 mins (run up, jog down to recover)	Strength training and stretch	Rest or yoga	Run 45 mins (with as few walk breaks as possible)*
Hill training 30 mins (run up, jog down to recover)	Strength training and stretch	Rest or yoga	Run 60 mins (with as few walk breaks as possible)
Hill training 30 mins (run up, jog down to recover)	Strength training and stretch	Rest or yoga	Run 65 mins (with as few walk breaks as possible)
Hill training 30 mins (run up, jog down to recover)	Strength training and stretch	Rest or yoga	Run 70 mins (with as few walk breaks as possible)

If you want to get faster over longer distances, try the following:

One weekly threshold session to increase your fitness levels – try blocks of 4 minutes at a speed that pushes you to the edge of discomfort with 4 minutes of recovery (see the 10-km training plan for examples of threshold sessions). As you get fitter, the threshold blocks can increase in duration. Only do this type of session once a week, as it is strenuous.

REGISTER FOR PARKRUN

It's worth signing up for parkrun (www.parkrun.org.uk), a timed weekly 5-km run which takes place in parks nationwide every Saturday morning. It's a free event, and you simply need to register online, then turn up and run. Every run is timed and emailed to you regularly. This will encourage you to push harder to get a faster time.

THE BIGGER PICTURE

Good nutrition and sleep are crucial if you want to improve your running. There's no point trying to push yourself harder on a run if you haven't slept for more than 4 hours or you've barely eaten anything all day. Remember that sleep will help your body to recover in between runs, while good nutrition will provide the fuel your body needs for energy.

STRONGER MEANS FITTER

Regular strength training will also help you improve your running. This doesn't mean lifting heavy weights, but working on leg strength is a good place to start. Body weight squats will strengthen the quadriceps (front thighs), and static and walking lunges will strengthen the hamstrings (rear thighs) and glutes (bottom). Don't neglect your core. Your core is the mid-section of the body and consists of muscles that support you and help hold you upright while you run. A weak core can lead to muscle imbalances, poor running technique and injury. Exercises like the plank and side plank are perfect for improving core strength.

It's also worth improving your balance. When you run, you are literally hopping from one foot to the other. Some single leg squats are ideal. Do them twice a week, ideally doing two or three sets of ten on each side.

Strengthen your glutes, as weak glutes can mean that your knee will start to twist inwards during running, which changes the forces and angle going down through your leg, putting stress on different areas of the lower body. Exercises like lunges, bridges and dirty dog will help. (Visit www.chrismacfitness.com for exercise demonstrations.)

RUNNING TECHNIQUE

When you run, aim to run tall, with shoulders positioned above your hips and your upper body having a slight lean forward from your hips. Imagine a thread pulling your head upwards. Try not to clench your fists as this can create tension in the upper body.

Running coach Nick Anderson from RunningWithUs says: 'There are so many mixed and confusing messages within the running industry regarding technique, but having a lighter foot plant and running with a mid-foot strike is definitely quicker and more efficient. Changes to technique can take time, requiring many months of specific exercises, drills and hard work.'

However, in an effort to keep things simple, Anderson recommends the following:

- Try to keep your hips high and retain good posture
- Have a slight forward lean almost as though you are falling forwards. This will enable gravity to tow you along
- Ideally your foot will land under you rather than ahead. This may require you to reduce your strike slightly but it should feel good when running tall and with a slight forward lean
- Try all of the above, but keep it natural

Anderson concludes: 'Our mantra is "up, light and tall". Think about this each time you run.'

RUNNING UPHILL

When running uphill, shorten your stride and take smaller steps, but don't slouch. Stay upright and propel yourself with your arms. Keep your elbows at a 90-degree angle.

RUNNING DOWNHILL

Downhill running can be painful on the shins and knees if you try to slow your pace. Try to go with the decline rather than braking. Don't lean backwards. Bend slightly forwards and try not to land on your heel.

TREADMILL RUNNING TECHNIQUE

- Don't run too close to the console, as you won't have much room to use your arms and you'll be inclined to pump them across your body, which causes unnecessary upper body rotation and can lead to stiffness in the upper back.
- Keep your head up and try not to spend too much time looking down at the console. Otherwise you may get pain in the neck or back.
- When you do look down, try to drop your eyes and not your head.
- Keep your shoulders back and chest up to open up the ribcage and allow you to get as much oxygen into your lungs as possible.
- Lift your knees so that your lower legs aren't doing all the work.

INCREASING THE DISTANCE

If you want to get better at distance running, complete one to two longer runs each week, adding no more than a mile each time. Your pace should be one that allows you to continue for long periods of time relatively comfortably. You would be able to have a full conversation if you were running with someone else. If you are unable to talk, then slow down. If you are wearing a heart rate monitor, you can monitor your heart rate more closely. You want to be working at around 70 to 80 per cent of your maximum heart rate (to work out your maximum heart rate, deduct your age from 220).

It's easy to fall into the trap of making every run a long run when you want to improve at distance running. This is not necessary and can lead to overtraining and injury. So long as you have a consistent weekly running schedule, your stamina will improve. On other running days, you could do a threshold run to improve your fitness. Harder runs should be shorter; easier paced runs can be longer. It's hard to be specific about total mileage per week, as it depends what distance you're training for. But broadly speaking, if you're training for a half-marathon, aim to run around 30 miles per week in total. Build up to this very gradually if you are a new runner – it can take up to 16 weeks to train for a half-marathon.

AT A GLANCE

- Increase volume gradually
- Build up from 5 km to 10 km with a structured training plan
- If running a 10-km race, reduce volume in the last two weeks
- To get faster, run with faster runners and join a running club
- Sign up for parkrun to get your weekly 5-km times recorded
- Do strengthening exercises regularly to improve muscle strength
- Check your running technique carefully
- Don't overdo the long runs

" My greatest running achievement to date has to be completing my first 10 km for charity without stopping. "

FAYE ANDREWS, OSTEOPATH

Chapter 11

CHOOSING AND PREPARING FOR YOUR FIRST RACE

CHOOSING YOUR FIRST RACE

Once you've become a regular runner, you may want to take part in a running event. On entering a race, you'll probably experience a renewed sense of enthusiasm. Having a specific distance to train for and a deadline is a great motivator.

It's normal to start with smaller distances like 5 km (3.12 miles) and 10 km (6.25 miles), but it's not uncommon to start with a half-marathon (21 km or 13.1 miles).

For a distance like a half-marathon, your longest run will need to be about 2 hours before race day. It would take most new runners around eight to ten weeks to train for a 5 km and around ten to 12 weeks to train for a 10 km, depending on your fitness levels. It would take most people around 12 to 16 weeks to train for a half-marathon and around 16 to 20 weeks to train for a full-marathon.

REASONS TO ENTER A RACE

- Better focus – it offers a fixed deadline for being able to run a certain distance
- Greater motivation – it gives you the incentive to get out and run
- Social interaction – you can train with friends
- Personal achievement – you'll get a great sense of achievement on race day when you collect your medal
- Improved confidence – knowing you can complete a certain distance can boost self-esteem
- Run for a good cause – you can raise money for charity

CHOOSE YOUR RACE CAREFULLY

Think about the type of race that would suit you. Consider the terrain you prefer to run on. If you prefer flat tarmac, an off-road muddy trail race could be your idea of hell. If you find flat urban surroundings boring, and you love the countryside, a trail race could be perfect.

Check the profile of the course first to see how challenging it is. If you choose a route with hills, you'll need to do some hill running.

Consider how far you want to travel to your race. If it's a local race, you may be grateful for a shorter journey home. If it's a race that involves extensive travel, you may want to book a hotel near the start line. Do this promptly, as demand (and prices) will be high.

To find a race, visit www.racebookuk.co.uk.

BIG OR SMALL?

It's worth considering the differences between small and large races. Larger races with more participants can be very crowded – but they tend to attract larger crowds, so you'll get great support. However, a crowded course means you'll either get stuck behind slower runners or have to weave past them, which can add distance to your run and be quite draining, especially near the end. If you're one of the slower runners, there will be lots of people passing you. If this happens, it's best to stay to the left-hand side. Large races can have a better atmosphere, but you'll probably have to queue longer for toilets and at the baggage collection (most races have a baggage drop-off point where you can leave personal items before the race to collect afterwards). Public transport to and from the race can also be very crowded.

Smaller races are more intimate, with fewer crowds to cheer you on. Smaller events organised by local running clubs can be very friendly, but some parts of the course can be quite empty, with only a handful of other runners around you. If you prefer to run in quieter surroundings, a smaller race could be a good choice.

RACING ABROAD

Racing abroad has become an increasingly popular way for runners to combine a holiday with their passion and is a great way to explore a new destination. While it can be a lot of fun, there are some key points to consider: the climate being one of them.

If you are going to be racing in a very hot country then it would be ideal to train in hot weather conditions, which is not always possible in the UK. But you could choose an autumn race and train through the summer, which will go some way towards getting you used to running in hot weather. If it's a country where temperatures will be cold, training in the UK during the winter months would be ideal, as you can not only get used to the cold but also try out your winter running wardrobe and make sure you have enough layers to keep you warm.

It's also worth considering how much travel is involved – if you're taking part in a longer race like a half-marathon or marathon, allow at least three days to recover from your journey before race day. Make a list of running kit to take with you before you go, as you may not be able to replace any forgotten items when you get there. Items to pack when racing abroad include:

- Vaseline
- Imodium
- Waist belt (to store energy gels, keys, etc.)
- Water bottle
- Sports bra
- Running kit for hot and cold weather
- Running socks
- A bin liner – to keep you warm at the start line
- Running shoes – an obvious item but surprisingly easy to forget!
- Blister plasters
- Safety pins to attach your race number
- Race pack and race number
- Course map and directions to the start line
- Energy gels, bars and energy drinks
- GPS watch

LOCAL FOOD

Research the local area, including how close your hotel is to the start and finish line and what cafes, restaurants and shops exist nearby (a local pharmacy is always a blessing).

Before you choose a location for your overseas race, have a think about what food is likely to be available. If you have a sensitive stomach, a location known for exotic dishes may present your digestive system with a few challenges!

PREPARING FOR YOUR FIRST RACE

You've signed up for your first challenge. Now what? The first piece of advice is to plan your training schedule. Your training needs to have a weekly structure. To get race fit, even if you're simply looking to 'get round' rather than complete the race in a specific time, the experience will be much more enjoyable if you train regularly. Get into a regular habit of going out for a run three times a week. Identify the gaps in your diary when you can run. If time is tight, try to build running into your day. For example, if you commute to work, change into your running kit and jump off the train a few stops earlier, completing your run on the way home.

Save longer runs for your days off, when you have more time. Remember: work-day runs don't need to be long. A threshold run or an out-and-back run that lasts 20 minutes will be fine. Short runs all add up.

Don't overdo your distance. It's a common myth that, if you're doing a race, you need to run the entire distance in training. If you're running 10 km, run up to 9 km in training. If you're doing a half-marathon (13.1 miles), run up to 10 miles. The crowd support on race day will get you through those last few miles. Provided you've run regularly, you will be fit enough.

It's also a myth that you need to run every day. Three times a week is fine. Make one run your longest, where you gradually build up mileage or time, and do two shorter, more intense sessions.

Although it's important to get into a regular routine when preparing for a race, it's also crucial to not overdo it. Every fourth week, have an easier recovery week. This means reducing volume on your longest run and maybe taking out one of your weekly runs, perhaps swapping it for an extra yoga class, or some light stretching. Remember to always stretch at the end of every run.

AT A GLANCE

- Think about whether you'd prefer trail or road races
- Check the course profile before you enter
- Do some hill training if your race contains hills
- If racing abroad, build in adequate time to recover from travel
- Make a list of items to take with you abroad
- Research the local area if it's new to you
- Plan your runs and write them in your diary
- Don't run the entire race distance in training

" Being a runner really makes you
feel invincible – I feel that as long
as I can run I'm alive and kicking! "

LORRAINE VOISEY, CARDIAC REHAB
SPECIALIST NURSE, MARATHON RUNNER

Chapter 12

RACE-DAY TACTICS

You've trained for the big day and it's here. You may feel a mixture of emotions – nerves, excitement, happiness and fear. This is normal. You're doing something you've never done before, so you're bound to feel some trepidation. However, the more you can plan ahead, the more smoothly things will go on race day. The night before the race, get your running kit and race pack containing your race number ready. Lay your kit out on the bed. If you're not sure what the weather will be like the next day, prepare two sets of kit. Have a few extra layers like a running jacket ready. Pin your race number on your top to save you doing it on race day while hunting around for safety pins.

  If the race is timed, there will be a timing chip either on the back of your race number, or it will be included separately in the race pack to attach to the laces of one of your shoes. Most race packs will have photo demonstrations of how to attach your timing chip. Again, do it the night before to make sure you don't forget.

  Get your energy gels and water bottle ready and leave them by the front door. If you wear a sports watch, make sure it's fully charged. Take a bin liner, with holes at the sides for your arms, to keep you warm while you wait for the race to start. (It can be easily discarded once you set off.)

  Make sure you know where the baggage drop-off point and start line are located. Plan how you'll get there. If you're planning to drive, find out where the nearest car parks are to the start line and how long it will take you to walk from the car park to the start line. If you're taking public transport, check train or bus times in advance and plan your journey, making sure there's no weekend engineering works on the trains that could affect your travel plans.

When you received your race pack, you would probably have received a sticker with your race number on and a carrier bag to store your personal items at the baggage drop-off area. You may want to pack a spare top and tracksuit bottoms in this bag to change into after the race to stop you getting cold on the way home.

Your race day nutrition strategy is well worth practising in advance. If you're doing a short race like a 5 km or a 10 km, you won't need to take gels or energy drinks. You may want to carry water for your own peace of mind, but all races will have water stations at regular intervals.

If you are doing a longer race like a half-marathon or marathon, you'll want to carry water, possibly also a waist belt containing two or three energy gels.

Only take gels or drinks you have already tested in training to avoid having an upset stomach. During the race, supporters may try to hand you sweets. Don't be tempted to eat anything new. The same goes for your pre-race breakfast. Try to eat your normal pre-run breakfast at the time you'd normally eat it before a run.

If you're doing a long race and you're worried about 'runner's trots', take Imodium Instants about 20 minutes before the start (they can be taken without water).

Plan and prepare, so that you're ready for race day, and you'll enjoy the experience so much more.

AT A GLANCE

- Read your race pack well in advance and again the night before the race
- Get your kit ready and plan for all weathers
- Remember to attach your timing chip to your shoe
- Plan how you'll get to the race and where you'll park
- Find out how near the start line is to your parking spot
- Practise your nutrition strategy in training
- Don't eat anything new on race day

" Running marathons makes you believe that you can achieve anything that you set out to. "

ANTHONY DURKIN, MANAGER, RUNNER

Chapter 13

GOING THE DISTANCE

It may sound like a dream to even think about running a marathon (26.2 miles or 42 km), but one day the subject may come up. It could be a random conversation with friends, or someone may ask if you've ever run one before. Completing a marathon can be a life-changing experience, and it may well give you the confidence to accomplish many other things in life.

Any healthy person (regardless of size or age) can run a marathon if they respect the distance. If you turn on the TV on the last Sunday in April, you'll see the evidence. Marathons don't discriminate by size, age or gender. But if you don't commit to the training, it won't be a pleasant experience and you may not even make it to the start line. But if you are genuinely prepared to train properly, then you stand a good chance of achieving your goal.

CAREFUL CONSIDERATION

Here's what you should know before you sign up for a marathon. The training will dominate at least four months of your life. Take a careful look at your work–life balance before you enter. If life is already very busy and stressful, adding more stress at this point may not be a good idea. When you are marathon training, you will think about little else. You'll either be running, eating for your next long run, stretching, planning your running schedule or talking about the marathon. You'll probably dream about it, too. It's scary, exciting, challenging and great fun. You'll feel alive and it can be a wonderful experience, but you need to be sure you are truly able to invest the time and effort.

Consider your current fitness levels and be honest about where you are now. While most healthy people can run a marathon with the right training, it's important to know how much time and effort it will take to get you race fit. Most marathon plans will recommend 16 to 20 weeks of training (longer is better, as it allows for time out due to illness or injury). If you're doing a marathon in April, ideally you want to be capable of running up to 10 miles non-stop by Christmas. It's also highly beneficial to run a couple of half-marathons so that you have some experience of distance running.

RUNNING FOR A GOOD CAUSE

Think about your starting point. Jan McLoughlin, director general of PDSA, the UK's leading vet charity, decided to run the London Marathon for the first time in 2010. As the head of a major charity, she wanted to lead by example. Jan felt that if she was heading up a charity that regularly appealed to people to run marathons to fundraise, then she should go through that marathon journey and run one herself. But Jan was honest with herself. By her own admission, at the age of 48, Jan was unfit and overweight. She wasn't doing any exercise and had undergone some knee operations in the past for torn cartilages. She knew that she was a long way from being ready to run a marathon. 'I knew I needed to lose a lot of weight and make sure I was in the best of health before I did any running,' Jan recalls.

In October 2009 (six months before the marathon), Jan hired a personal trainer to help her lose weight and improve her strength.

She knew that if she had less weight to carry and her muscles were stronger, her chances of completing the marathon successfully would be vastly increased. She says: 'I spent the first few months building up my core strength and getting my eating and training habits aligned, so that I could see the weight loss and also had the energy to do something with it. I spent from October to December improving my fitness and started to run in January.'

Jan lost a total of 3 stone first and then decided it was time to start running. For added support, she joined a running club. This made a big difference. Jan says: 'There's always an excuse not to go out and run, but I always think I am going to let somebody down if I don't go out.' Jan went out running three times a week at first, eventually increasing it to four.

Despite turning her ankle at mile 17 of the marathon, Jan went on to complete the London Marathon in 5:08. Now she credits running with giving her more energy and has gone on to complete the London Marathon a further two times, knocking her time down to 4:47 on both occasions. To date she has raised over £50,000 for PDSA and has inspired her work colleagues to be active. 'It seems to have inspired a lot of much younger runners than me to take part and help raise funds for our charity,' Jan adds.

Her next goal is to run the London Marathon again in 2017, which is the centenary year of PDSA, with 100 runners joining her on the start line in PDSA vests.

Her advice for anyone wanting to run a marathon is to get your body strong to withstand the demands of distance running first. 'Think about where your sensitive points are,' Jan says. 'If it's your knees, ankles or your calves, build up gradually, get your diet right, too – you can't run a car with an empty tank. You've got to get the balance between your diet, your exercise and just build it up gradually.'

This is good advice. Before you start marathon training, see a physiotherapist or running coach, and get them to check your running style and look for any weaknesses or imbalances that can be addressed first. Get the support you need, like Jan did.

Jan's story demonstrates her commitment to putting in the effort that was needed to succeed.

FIND A REASON TO RUN

Consider what running a marathon means to you. Have a compelling reason to run one – whether it's to raise money for charity or to prove to yourself that you can do it.

If your motives are strong, it's simply a case of committing to the training. Contrary to popular belief, you can run a marathon on three or four good-quality runs per week (three is my preference), but I'd strongly advise following a structured training plan. Visit www.womensrunninguk.co.uk for marathon training plans for all abilities suitable for men and women.

TRAINING WEEK

During a typical training week, you should aim to do one long run, where you gradually increase time each week, one interval or threshold session and one shorter hill session. You can do the two shorter sessions on the treadmill, but your long run should ideally be outside, so that you get used to running in all weather conditions.

On non-running days, do a fourth cardio session on the cross-trainer. Go swimming or cycling if you don't have a cross-trainer. I'd also suggest two good-quality strength sessions per week, working on legs and core. A weekly or twice-weekly yoga class will be hugely beneficial.

Your longest run should be no more than 22 miles. The ideal range is between 18 and 21 miles. You don't need to run the full 26.2 miles in training, as this could mean you're already fatigued when you reach the start line. In any case, the crowd support will get you round the last 5 miles.

Do your longest run three weeks before race day. Wear the running kit you intend to wear on race day, to make sure it's comfortable. Test your energy gels and drinks beforehand.

After your longest run, reduce your mileage and the duration of your long runs. Drop your weekly volume of running by around 20 to 30 per cent. With two weeks left, reduce your training volume by around 50 to 70 per cent of your normal total. In the final week, just short runs of up to 30 minutes will be fine and make sure you rest in the last few days leading up to the marathon.

LOOK AFTER YOURSELF

During the last month, make a real effort to get more sleep. Eat well to fuel your long runs and avoid dieting or trying to lose weight at all costs.

After the marathon, have a sports massage within three days of the race and give yourself a few days off from any training. After a week of rest, some light jogging or a few easy sessions on the cross-trainer or a light swim or cycle should be fine and you can gradually ease back into training after a few weeks.

AT A GLANCE

- Establish your current starting point – how fit are you now?
- Make sure you have enough time to commit to training
- Have a compelling reason to run a marathon
- Build up training gradually – three runs a week is fine
- Cross-train to reduce injury risk
- Eat well, sleep more – don't diet
- Stretch, stretch and stretch!

" Since doing the marathon, I have
a more positive outlook on life.
The sense of accomplishment is
something I'll carry with me forever. "

GARY HEAD, PERSONAL TRAINER

Chapter 14

PAY IT FORWARD

You may be so inspired by what you've achieved that you'll be keen to share the benefits of running with others. If you have friends who want to start, you could help them get motivated by sharing your knowledge and experience.

To inspire others, you could set up your own running group and become a qualified running group leader. Anyone can do it: all you need is enthusiasm for running and a desire to help new runners get started.

You need to get a valid and recognised UKA licence to lead a group. To do this, you need to complete a one-day Run England course called the Leadership in Running Fitness qualification (which costs approx. £155) and then complete a DBS (Disclosure and Barring Service) check to register your running licence. The course takes place at locations nationwide and will show you how to deliver safe running sessions for people of all abilities. The course also covers goal-setting, warming up and cooling down, and common running injuries. For more information, visit the Run England website at www.runengland.org/leader.

After the course, you can set up your own running group, which can be as informal as taking six workmates out for a run or setting up your own website and arranging for your group to become affiliated and approved by Sport England (see Run England website for more information).

Another way to help others is to become a race marshal. This simply means pointing runners in the right direction during a race. parkrun (www.parkrun.org.uk) is always looking for volunteers, but so are many other race organisations. Simply contact the race organisers directly.

You could also become a race pacer and help others achieve their desired race times. Races with pacers cater for all abilities, so you don't have to be fast to do it. A 10-km race, for instance, may have pacers for 50 minutes, 60 minutes and 70 minutes.

FINAL THOUGHTS

You've proved you can run. You might have had a role model who helped you. If you know someone who doubts their ability to run, encourage them as much as you can. It might be a good time to dig out that running journal and see how far you've come. When you look back, you may be surprised by how much you've achieved.

RUNNING DIRECTORY

APPS

Active Goals – www.subthree.co.uk

Couch to 5K – www.nhs.uk/Livewell/c25k/Pages/couch-to-5k.aspx

MapMyRun – www.mapmyrun.com/routes/create

MyFitnessPal – www.myfitnesspal.com

Nike Run – http://secure-nikeplus.nike.com/plus

Pumatrac – http://global.puma.com/en/pumatrac

Runkeeper – www.runkeeper.com

Runtastic – www.runtastic.com

Strava – www.strava.com

RUNNING STORES

www.achillesheel.co.uk

www.asics.co.uk

www.decathlon.co.uk

www.profeet.co.uk

www.runnersneed.com

www.runandbecome.com

www.sweatshop.co.uk

www.upandrunning.co.uk

ONLINE RETAILERS

www.milletsports.co.uk/running

www.prodirectrunning.com

www.sportsshoes.com

www.wiggle.co.uk/run

TO FIND A RACE

www.active.com

www.goodrunguide.co.uk/racefinder.asp

www.mynextrun.com

www.racebookuk.co.uk

www.runningdiary.co.uk

www.runnersworld.co.uk/events

http://scottishrunningguide.com

USEFUL RUNNING WEBSITES

www.fetcheveryone.com

www.marathontalk.com

www.parkrun.org.uk

www.mensrunninguk.co.uk

www.runengland.org

www.runnersworld.co.uk

http://running.competitor.com

www.therunningbug.co.uk

www.runlounge.com

www.thisgirlcan.co.uk

www.veggierunners.com

www.womensrunninguk.co.uk

RACES

(All information was correct at the time of going to press – please note, race sponsors and dates can sometimes be subject to change)

Adidas Silverstone Half Marathon, March – www.adidashalfmarathon.com

ASICS Greater Manchester Marathon, April –
www.greatermanchestermarathon.com

Bacchus Marathon, Dorking, September – www.eventstolive.co.uk

Bath Half-Marathon, March – http://bathhalf.co.uk/entries

Baxters River Ness 5K Fun Run, Inverness, September –
www.lochnessmarathon.com

Beachy Head Marathon, October – www.visiteastbourne.com

Blackpool Marathon, April –
www.marathonrunnersdiary.com/races/uk-marathons/blackpool-marathon.php

Bournemouth Half-Marathon, October – www.run-bmf.com/?marathon_eventinfo

Brathay Windermere Marathon, May – www.brathaywindermeremarathon.org.uk

Brighton Marathon, April – www.brightonmarathonweekend.co.uk

Bristol Half Marathon, September – www.runbristol.com

British Heart Foundation Hyde Park Run, London, October –
www.bhf.org.uk/get-involved-events

RUNNING DIRECTORY

Brooks Fleet Half Marathon, March – fleethalfmarathon.com
Bupa London 10,000, May – www.london10000.co.uk

Cancer Research UK Race for Life Pretty Muddy, various dates around the UK –
    www.raceforlife.cancerresearchuk.org
Cardiff Half Marathon, October – www.cardiffhalfmarathon.co.uk
Causeway Coast Marathon, County Antrim, September –
    www.26extreme.com/eventscalendar.aspx
Chester Half Marathon, May – www.activeleisureevents.co.uk/half-marathon
Croydon Half Marathon, May – www.croydonhalf.co.uk
The Color Run UK, series of 5-km races in London, Manchester, Birmingham,
    Belfast, Sunderland and Brighton, typically from June to September –
    www.thecolorrun.co.uk

Ealing Half Marathon, September – www.ealinghalfmarathon.com
Edinburgh Marathon, May – www.edinburgh-marathon.com
English Half Marathon, September – www.run-ehm.com

Forest of Dean Autumn Half-Marathon, September –
    www.forestofdean-halfmarathon.co.uk

Garmin Kingston Run Challenge (8.2, 16 or 26.2 miles), October –
    www.humanrace.co.uk/events/running/kingston-run-challenge
Great Welsh Marathon, April –
    www.active.com/llanelli-carmarthenshire/running/distance-running-races/
    great-welsh-marathon-and-half-marathon-2016

Hastings Half Marathon, March – www.hastings-half.co.uk/article.php/33/race_information
Heroes Run – www.heroesrun.org.uk

Ikano Robin Hood Half-Marathon, September – www.robinhoodhalfmarathon.co.uk
Inverness Half-Marathon, March – www.invernesshalfmarathon.co.uk
Isle of Wight Marathon, Cowes, October – www.rydeharriers.co.uk

Leeds Abbey Dash, Leeds, November – www.ageuk.org.uk
Lidl Kingston Breakfast Run (8.2, 16.2 or 20.1 miles), March –
    www.humanrace.co.uk/events/running/breakfast-run

The Major Series, various dates, 5-km and 10-km obstacle races – www.majorseries.com
MBNA Chester Marathon, October – www.activeleisureevents.co.uk/marathon

Milton Keynes Half Marathon, March – www.mkrun.co.uk

Milton Keynes Marathon, May – www.mkmarathon.com/mk-marathon-2

Morrisons Great Run Series (Great Birmingham Run, Great Edinburgh Run, Great North Run, Great Scottish Run, Great South Run, Great Yorkshire Run) – distances include 2 km, 5 km, 10 miles and 13.1 miles – www.greatrun.org

MoRun (5 km), November – www.mo-running.com/cardiff

Pharmalink Maidenhead Half Marathon, September – www.purplepatchrunning.com

Perkins Great Eastern Run (half-marathon), October – www.perkinsgreateasternrun.co.uk

Plusnet Yorkshire Marathon, October – www.theyorkshiremarathon.com

The Poppy Run 5K, venues nationwide, October and November – www.poppy-run.com

Pride Run 10K, London, August – www.pride10k.org

Race for Life 5 km series, venues nationwide throughout the summer – http://raceforlife.cancerresearchuk.org/index.html

Race for Life half-marathon (women only), October, Lee Valley – http://raceforlife.cancerresearchuk.org/types-of-event/half-marathon/index.html

Race for Life Women's Only Marathon, October – raceforlife.cancerresearchuk.org/types-of-event/marathon/index.html

Race Your Pace Half, Windsor, February – www.marathonandahalf.co.uk/Race-your-pace-half-marathon.html

Richmond Park Marathon, May – www.richmondparkmarathon.co.uk

Rock 'n' Roll Dublin Half Marathon, August – www.ie.competitor.com/dublin

Rock 'n' Roll Liverpool Marathon, Half-Marathon or 5K, May – www.runrocknroll.com/liverpool

Royal Parks Half Marathon, October – www.royalparkshalf.com

Run For All Leeds 10K, July – www.runforall.com/10k/leeds

Saucony Cambridge Half Marathon, February – www.onestepbeyond.org.uk/cambridge-half-marathon-info-request.php

Shakespeare Marathon, April – www.shakespearemarathon.org.uk

Spartan Race (obstacle races), various dates – www.uk.spartanrace.com

Standard Chartered Great City Race, July – www.cityrace.co.uk

Surrey Badger Half Marathon, July – www.eventstolive.co.uk

Sure Run to the Beat 10K, September – www.runtothebeat.co.uk/event

Tough Mudder, various dates, 10–12-mile obstacle races – www.toughmudder.co.uk

Virgin Money London Marathon, April – www.virginmoneylondonmarathon.com/en-gb
Vitality British 10K, London, July – www.thebritish10klondon.co.uk
Vitality Hackney Half Marathon – www.runhackney.com
Vitality Liverpool Half Marathon, March –
    www.btrliverpool.com/#!liverpool-half-marathon/cjg9
Vitality North London Half Marathon, March – www.northlondonhalf.com
Vitality Oxford Half Marathon, October – www.oxfordhalf.co.uk
Vitality Reading Half Marathon, April – www.readinghalfmarathon.com

Windsor & Eton Half Marathon, Dorney Lake, March –
    www.halfmarathonlist.co.uk/dorney-lake-half-marathon.php
Women's Running 10K Race Series, typically from May to September,
    locations nationwide – womensrunninguk.co.uk

USEFUL NUTRITION WEBSITES
    Beat Eating Disorders – www.b-eat.co.uk
    British Nutrition Foundation – www.nutrition.org.uk
    HealthStatus – www.healthstatus.com
        (has online calculators to work out your BMI and daily calorie needs)
    Vegetarian Society – www.vegsoc.org
    Weight Loss Resources – www.weightlossresources.co.uk